6. 3 - 24

Oxford,

CLINICS
IN
ENDOCRINOLOGY
AND
METABOLISM

CLINICS IN ENDOCRINOLOGY AND METABOLISM

VOLUME 11/NUMBER 3
NOVEMBER 1982

DISEASES OF SEX AND SEXUALITY

John Bancroft, MD, MRCP, FRCPsych
Guest Editor

W. B. Saunders Company Ltd London · Philadelphia · Toronto

W. B. Saunders Company Ltd: 1 St Anne's Road
Eastbourne, East Sussex BN21 3UN

West Washington Square
Philadelphia, PA 19105, USA

1 Goldthorne Avenue
Toronto, Ontario M8Z 5T9, Canada

Cedro 512
Mexico 4, DF Mexico

9 Waltham Street
Artarmon, NSW 2064, Australia

Ichibancho Central Bldg, 22-1 Ichibancho,
Chiyoda-ku, Tokyo 102, Japan

ISSN 0300-595X

Clinics in Endocrinology and Metabolism is published three times each year by W. B. Saunders
Company Ltd. Subscription price is £21.50 per annum.

The editor of this publication is Dr Barend ter Haar, W. B. Saunders Company Ltd, 1 St
Anne's Road, Eastbourne, East Sussex BN21 3UN.

Printed at The Lavenham Press Ltd, Lavenham, Suffolk, England.

Contributors to This Issue

JOHN BANCROFT, MD, MRCP, FRCPsych, Honorary Senior Lecturer, Department of Psychiatry, University of Edinburgh; Honorary Clinical Consultant, Lothian Health Board; MRC Reproductive Biology Unit, Centre for Reproductive Biology, Edinburgh EH3 9EW.

GRAHAM D. BURROWS, MD, ChB, DPM, FRANZCP, FRCPsych, First Assistant and Reader, Department of Psychiatry, University of Melbourne, Royal Melbourne Hospital, Parkville, Victoria 3050, Australia; Chairman, Royal Melbourne Hospital Department of Psychiatry.

JULIAN M. DAVIDSON, PhD, Professor of Physiology, Stanford University, Stanford, CA 94305, USA.

LORRAINE DENNERSTEIN, MB, BS, PhD, DPM, MRANZCP, Senior Lecturer, Department of Psychiatry, University of Melbourne, Royal Melbourne Hospital, Parkville, Victoria 3050, Australia; Director, Psychosomatic Gynaecology Clinic, Royal Melbourne Hospital.

CHRISTOPHER G. FAIRBURN, MA, MPhil, MRCPsych, Research Psychiatrist, University of Oxford, Department of Psychiatry, Warneford Hospital, Oxford OX3 7JX.

CHARLES FISHER, MD, PhD, Emeritus Clinical Professor of Psychiatry, Mount Sinai School of Medicine, New York, NY 10029, USA.

WALTER J. GREENLEAF, Graduate Research Assistant, Department of Physiology, Stanford University, Stanford, CA 94305, USA.

GÖTZ KOCKOTT, MD, Lecturer, Technische Universität München, Psychiatrische Klinik und Poliklinik v.d. Isar, Möhlstrasse 26, 8000 München 80, FR Germany.

MARIE KWAN, PhD, Research Fellow, Department of Physiology, Stanford University, Stanford, CA 94305, USA.

DAVID K. McCULLOCH, MRCP, Research Fellow, University Hospital, Queen's Medical Centre, Nottingham.

HEINO F. L. MEYER-BAHLBURG, Dr.rer.nat., Associate Professor of Clinical Psychology, Department of Psychiatry, Columbia University College of Physicians and Surgeons, 722 West 168th Street, New York, NY 10032, USA; Research Scientist, New York State Psychiatric Institute; Pediatric Behavioural Endocrinologist in Psychiatry Service, The Presbyterian Hospital, New York.

VÁCLAV MICHAL, MD, DrSc(med), Clinical Scientific Officer, Cardiovascular Research Centre and Department of Surgery, Institute for Clinical and Experimental Medicine, Vídeňská 800, 146 22 Prague-Krč, Czechoslovakia.

K. M. PIRKE, Dr.med.habil., Senior Investigator, Max-Planck-Institut für Psychiatrie, Abteilung für Klinische Chemie, Kraepelinstrasse 10, 8000 München 40, FR Germany.

SHIRLEY G. RATCLIFFE, MB, BS, FRCPE, Consultant Paediatrician, Medical Research Council Clinical and Population Cytogenetics Unit, Western General Hospital, Crewe Road, Edinburgh EH4 2XU, and Royal Hospital for Sick Children, Edinburgh.

DIANA J. SANDERS; PhD, Postdoctoral Research Fellow, Psychology Department, University of Canterbury, Christchurch, New Zealand; *formerly* Research Psychologist, MRC Reproductive Biology Unit, Edinburgh.

RAUL C. SHIAVI, MD, Profesor of Psychiatry, Mount Sinai School of Medicine, New York, NY 10029, USA; Director, Human Sexuality Program, Mount Sinai Medical Center, Attending; Mount Sinai Hospital.

GORM WAGNER, MD, Associate Professor, Department of Medical Physiology B, The Panum Institute, University of Copenhagen, Copenhagen, Denmark.

F. C. WU, MRCP, Senior Registrar in Endocrinology, Department for Endocrine and Metabolic Diseases, Western General Hospital, Crewe Road, Edinburgh EH4 2XU.

Table of Contents

RECENT ISSUES

FORTHCOMING ISSUE

Foreword

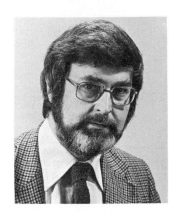

In the field of medical sexology, fashions have certainly changed over the past 50 years. In the 1930s much attention was paid to physical causes and methods of treatment, many of which now seem absurd. This was followed by a swing to psychogenic causation and emphasis on psychological methods of treatment. The pendulum is now swinging back. In some respects, it may be going too far, but there are now good reasons to think that the interaction between physical and psychological factors is at last beginning to receive proper attention.

A combination of this more balanced approach with the rapid development of new techniques and investigation of physical and biological factors promises rapid progress in our understanding over the next few years. Some of the current steps in this direction are covered in this issue.

The first four chapters are concerned with the relationship between hormones and sexuality in the adult. Julian Davidson's chapter provides a thorough review of our present knowledge of hormones and sexuality in men, whilst Karl Pirke and Götz Kockott provide some additional research evidence in this area. Diana Sanders and I consider the relevance of the menstrual cycle to the sexuality of women and the extremely intriguing question of the role of androgens in female sexuality. Lorraine Dennerstein and Graham Burrows consider the importance of hormones in women following the menopause or surgical removal of their ovaries. There are more questions than answers in these four chapters, but it is reasonable to conclude that we are beginning to fill in a complex jigsaw puzzle.

Chapters 5 and 6 are concerned with developmental aspects. Heino Meyer-Bahlburg reviews our present knowledge of the hormonal control of sexual differentiation and its relevance to sexual orientation. Shirley Ratcliffe discussed the recently initiated prospective developmental studies of children with sex chromosome abnormalities.

Chapters 7 and 8 are concerned specifically with problems of penile erection. Gorm Wagner considers the possible physiological mechanisms involved in erection and how they can go wrong. This much neglected aspect of physiology is at last receiving the attention it deserves. The importance of vascular disease as a cause of erectile impotence is being increasingly recognized. Václav Michal presents an impressive body of data to persuade us that peripheral arterial disease, affecting penile vessels, is not only a common cause of erectile failure, but a potentially treatable one. This field is certainly in its infancy, but there can be little doubt of its potential importance.

The last three chapters focus on diabetes and sexual function. Christopher Fairburn and his colleagues provide a broad review of sexual dysfunction in male diabetics. Raul Schiavi and Charles Fisher provide a balanced, critical and much needed review of the diagnostic value of measuring nocturnal penile tumescence in such cases. I conclude the issue with a brief review of sexual problems in diabetic women.

In most of these chapters, the need to understand psychological reactions to physical processes, or in other words to apply the psychosomatic model, will be very evident. I believe that you will find this international collection a good sample of modern thinking in research into diseases of sexuality.

JOHN BANCROFT

1

Hormonal Replacement and Sexuality in Men

JULIAN M. DAVIDSON
MARIE KWAN
WALTER J. GREENLEAF

INTRODUCTION

Though castration has been used to manipulate the behaviour of domestic animals and men, literally for millenia, the scientific study of androgen replacement therapy for hyposexuality is still in its infancy. This is all the more surprising since a great volume of research in the last half-century has established the vital importance of testicular androgen in maintaining sexual function in infrahuman mammals of all species which have been studied, as well as in animals of other orders. In fact, while androgen treatment for hypogonadism is common practice in modern medicine, it was only in 1979/80 that adequately controlled studies demonstrating the reactivation of sexual behaviour with testosterone replacement therapy in hypogonadal men were first published. Hopefully these studies were only the opening salvos in an impending barrage of investigation on the relation ships between androgen and male sexuality. The many questions which remain to be answered can be arranged in two classes: parametric and mechanistic.

Parametric issues, involving mostly dose-response relationships, are of more than simple practical interest since, along with their role in establishing rational clinical approaches to replacement therapy, they also bear on mechanisms of action. Thus, how androgen works on human behaviour cannot be studied rationally until we know exactly which behavioural patterns or components thereof are affected. The latency from administration of androgen to onset of sexual effect, for instance, and particularly the differences (if such exist) in relative latency between different components of sexual behaviour, are most relevant to constructing hypotheses on how and where the hormone acts. This approach has been utilized in studies on sexual behaviour in experimental animals using specific tests for erectile, ejaculatory and motivational components of copulatory behaviour (Davidson, Gray and Smith, 1979, 1981). It should be applicable with at least equal benefit to men.

This chapter will first consider the use of different androgens for whatever purpose replacement therapy is utilized, and will then go on to

Clinics in Endocrinology and Metabolism — Vol. 11, No. 3, November 1982.
0300-595X/82/11.03/599 $03.00 © 1982 W. B. Saunders Company Ltd

discuss sexuality in castrates, to present the recent double-blind studies, and to consider parametric data; finally, possible mechanisms of the action of androgen on sex behaviour will be discussed. To a considerable extent this chapter is an update and critical appraisal of the relevant sections of Bancroft's excellent review of human sexual endocrinology (1980), since we agree on the nature of the major issues in current research.

ANDROGEN REPLACEMENT THERAPY IN GENERAL

Androgen treatment is used (a) for pharmacological reasons (e.g. for metabolic effects in eugonadal subjects); (b) to replace functions other than sexual behaviour (e.g., normalization of secondary sexual characteristics, bone and nitrogen metabolism in hypogonadals); and (c) for maintenance of sexuality.

The testis is the source of almost all of the biologically potent androgen in a normal male, and it is most rational to treat castrated or hypogonadal men with the major testicular androgen testosterone (T). Unfortunately, this hormone is ineffective when administered parenterally or by mouth because of rapid inactivation by the liver, so replacement therapy has most often been practised by injection of long-acting esters of T (e.g., enanthate and cypionate) or oral administration of other synthetic androgens. In the former case, esterification of T slows its release into the circulation by increasing its solubility in lipid vehicles, while other molecular modifications have the effect of slowing metabolism by the liver. In the latter category of synthetic androgens the most commonly used in the USA, methyltestosterone and fluoxymesterone, are 17α-alkylated. This modification can result in abnormalities of liver function extending from mild cholestatic jaundice to rare cases of hepatoma and peliosis hepatis. While the esters have to be hydrolysed before effective action of androgen on cells, the 17α-alkylated derivatives appear to be active within the cell without modification. It is more difficult to monitor the activity of the latter (orally active) synthetics for assessment of the effectiveness of therapy, since blood levels have to be assayed using specific methods which are infrequently available, whereas commonly available T assays can be used for the T esters. (See Wilson and Griffin, 1980.)

In addition to the above-mentioned androgens another synthetic, mesterolone (1α-methyl-5α-androstan-17β-ol-3-one), is not prescribed in the USA but is often used elsewhere.

SEXUALITY IN CASTRATES

Determination of the effects of castration on sexuality at different ages is a matter of primary interest since it is generally assumed that the 'baseline' on which androgen acts is the level of sexuality found in the prepuberal castrate. Though we know little of the effects on sexuality of pubertal exposure to androgen, clinical data indicate that prepuberal hypogonadism is more difficult to treat with replacement therapy than is postpuberal hypogonadism (Money and Clopper, 1975). This discussion will concern only adult castrates. It should be noted that the 'baseline' androgen level in these individuals is not negligible, but there is no substantial information on the role of adrenal androgen in male sexuality, if any.

Though untold thousands of men have been castrated throughout history, it is remarkable how little reliable, detailed information is available on the potential or actual level of sexuality in castrates. In modern societies, castration has often been practised as a legal procedure, yet the literature is replete with grave doubts about the efficacy of castration as a treatment for sexual offenders (Heim and Hursch, 1979; Heim, 1981). Literary sources reinforce the notion that sexual function can be retained in castrates — even emasculated eunuchs! (Mitamura, 1970). After reviewing the early clinical writings on castration Kinsey, in his monumental work, argues strongly against a specific role of androgen in sexual function (Kinsey et al, 1953, pp. 738-745), claiming that castration has 'little or no effect on the sexual responsiveness of half or more of the males', and that the gradual decline in sexuality after castration was simply a manifestation of the general decline due to aging.

Since the Kinsey report there have been a number of surveys on the effects of legal castration on sexuality; they also report considerable retention of sexual function in castrates, sometimes for many years. However, as Heim shows (Heim and Hursch, 1979; Heim, 1981), the studies on castrates are rife with methodological weaknesses. These include the use of retrospective verbal report, often involving long-term memory; limitation of behavioural descriptions to vague terms like potency and libido, used without definition; the probable unreliability of many informants; the absence of attempts to assess the validity of data; the omission of statistical analysis and the lack of prospective studies. Nevertheless, some conclusions can be drawn from these less-than-optimal studies. There is little doubt that after castration sexual behaviour (operationally defined, for example, as activities leading to orgasm) is drastically reduced or completely suppressed in a high percentage of men. On the other hand, a far-from-negligible percentage of castrates retain a significant degree of sexual function. Reports vary from 37 per cent complete loss of 'sexual response' (Wolf, 1934) to 90 per cent 'desexualized' (Sturup, 1979). No systematic attempts have been made to assess the contribution to the sexual outcome of factors such as preoperative level of sexuality, aging, psychological effects of the surgery, as well as problems associated with legal or medical reasons for the surgery. It is also not clear what sexuality is really like for the remaining 10 to 63 per cent of castrates who are purportedly not 'desexualized'. All we seem to know is that these castrates engage in sexual activity of some kind, but they could be doing so for reasons other than sexual desire or pleasure (e.g., to satisfy their partners or self image). Thus castrates may have isolated retention of erectile function. In fact a recent report on 'legal' castrates apparently indicates that 50 per cent of 38 men castrated 3 to 5 years previously responded to erotic film with 'full' erections (Eibl, 1978, cited by Heim and Hursch, 1979). But what degree of sexual desire, enjoyment, satisfaction and orgasm is retained? The reviews of this literature (Beach, 1948; Kinsey et al, 1953; Sturup, 1969; Heim and Hursch, 1979; Heim, 1981) are virtually silent on these questions so vital to assessing the nature and extent of the castrated man's sexuality and therefore the role of hormone replacement therapy for hypogonadism.

THE CATEGORIES AND ELEMENTS OF SEXUALITY

By this point the reader may be feeling some disquiet relative to terminology and assessment of sexual function. Since the authors share that disquiet, a brief discussion of this issue follows. It is fairly obvious that the term sexuality covers a large conglomerate of human behaviour and experience too complex ever to be studied usefully without due regard to its constituents. Unfortunately, however, there is no agreement as to what exactly these constituents are and what they define. Therefore we shall attempt only to present operational definitions just general enough to reflect the most common usage, yet just precise enough to be of some use. In doing this we distinguish between (a) those categories of sexuality which dominate our thinking about sexuality: libido and potency; and (b) *elements* of sexuality: individual behaviours, capacities or cognitive acts which are component parts of libido and potency (see Figure 1).

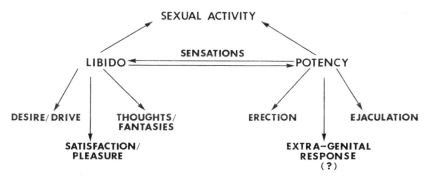

Figure 1. A simplified diagram depicting relationships between the categories of male sexuality required for sexual activity, libido and potency and the elements of which they consist. Inter-relationships are shown by arrows. Each of the elements can be used in assessment of sexuality, though more research is required to identify specific sexual patterns of extra-genital physiological response. 'Sensations' denotes perceptions of physiological sexual response; these participate in the postulated positive feedback relationship between libido and potency (see 'Behavioural mechanism of action of androgen').

Libido is, in our view, the sum of the affective-cognitive processes which result in the tendency to engage in sexual behaviour. It is the equivalent of the 'sexual motivation' of animal research. The elements of libido involve conscious events which reflect sexual 'interest', i.e. desire for sexual activity, expressed in increased sexual thoughts and fantasies. Related to these elements are those of enjoyment, pleasure or satisfaction derived from engaging in or thinking about sexual activity, as well as the importance the individual attributes to his/her sexuality. Potency is defined, for our purposes, as the capacity to respond to sexual stimuli (exogenous or endogenous) with physiological genitopelvic responses: primarily (a) erection and associated vasomotor activity, and (b) ejaculation and associated neuromuscular activity. The extragenital neural, vascular and muscular reactions are not included in this operational definition (though they may be in a future one) simply because patterns *specific* to sexual affect have not been clearly identified and utilized in sexual assessment.

Because of the interactions between libido and potency (Davidson, 1980) a true assessment of either can be made only when influences of the other are excluded. In the most studied species, the laboratory rat, a dose-related response of sexual motivation to T in the absence of genital sensation or erection is shown quantitatively by the increased frequency of mounting oestrous females following penile anaesthetization (Gray, Smith and Davidson, 1981). No very satisfactory quantitative measures exist for humans, but self-appraisal of intensity of sexual desire and frequency of thoughts or fantasies are used. The orgasmic altered state of consciousness (Davidson, 1980) should belong in the category of libido and can be assessed in terms of frequency, intensity and latency. In practice it is usually classed under potency because it is confused with ejaculation.

With the advent of the sexual psychophysiology laboratory potency could be measured in terms of latency to responding and amplitude and duration of response, when objective measurement is feasible. Since potency, as defined here, is strongly influenced by strength of libido, it is important to assess this category in circumstances devoid of sexually-arousing stimuli. A clear androgen-dependence of erections can be shown in rats under these circumstances by measuring reflex responses which occur in rhythmic clusters when the animal is restrained in a supine position (Hart, 1967; Davidson et al, 1978). Similarly in rats the androgen dependence of ejaculation in the absence of a sexual partner (and thus, presumably, of sexual arousal) is seen in the stimulation by T of spontaneous emission, which occurs on average once each 'night' (the light period, when the rat sleeps) (M. L. Stefanick and J. M. Davidson, 1982 unpublished observation). In the human, tests for potency isolated from libido influences are much more problematic; for example, nocturnal emissions are rare in the adult, and elicitation of orgasm in the laboratory presents obvious difficulties. As to erection, the best measure presently available is the recording of nocturnal penile tumescence (NPT) considered to be a measure of erectile potency uncontaminated by psychogenic factors (Karacan, 1982, but see Wasserman et al (1980) and Chapter 10 for caveats).

HORMONES AND SEXUALITY IN AGING MEN

Aging men have often been considered as potential recipients of androgen replacement therapy for hyposexuality. Do men become hypogonadal in aging if and when their sexual functioning declines? If so, is there a causal relationship between the low androgen level and the behavioural changes? Answers are available in the existing literature to the first question but not to the second. It is well established from numerous studies that a clear downward trend in sexual function in aging men (Kinsey, Pomeroy and Martin, 1948; Voerwoerdt, Pfeiffer and Wang, 1969a, b) is accompanied by a parallel decline in plasma T and an increase in gonadotrophin level (Vermeulen, Rubens and Verdonck, 1972; Baker et al, 1976; Stearns et al, 1976). The nature of the changes in sexual function and endocrinology have been reviewed recently (Davidson, Gray and Smith, 1982). It appears, though behaviourally sophisticated studies are rare, that all aspects of sexuality are affected by the aging decline, but variables reflecting libido show a lesser decline than potency, thus producing a libido-potency gap which can make the situation of the older man particularly difficult.

We have recently completed a study of hormones and sexuality in 220 ambulatory men aged 41 to 93 years, interviewed while visiting a hospital outpatient clinic to give blood samples for routine health checks or other testing purposes (Davidson et al, unpublished data 1982). Plasma was analysed for a variety of reproductive hormones and subjects were given a questionnaire dealing with various aspects of sexuality. As most of the other studies have found, total plasma T decreased, sex hormone binding globulin increased and consequently there was a greater decrease in free T level (calculated from total T and sex hormone binding protein activity) than in total T. Along with this there were rises in LH and FSH, but no change in oestradiol or prolactin levels.

Behavioural questionnaire data were scored on scales of 1 to 5, and a variety of statistical methods was used to study the possible relationship between hormonal and behavioural variables. Composite scores for libido (interest and thoughts or fantasies) and performance (activity and potency) were constructed by averaging responses to several questions. The decline in both sexes was most obvious in, men over 70 years (particularly performance) but was clearly present also in the seventh decade of life.

Table 1 shows that there were significant correlations between hormonal and behavioural (libido or performance) variables, as expected when a population of this size and age span is surveyed. A number of points in Table 1 are important to note. First, the significant correlations are of a low order, suggesting that the hormone-behaviour relationship is not very strong. Secondly, they affect performance variables more than libido. Thirdly, LH is better correlated than free T with behavioural measures, and total T is never so correlated. Perhaps most importantly, the correlations tend to diminish when they are run *within* decades of life, which eliminates most of the influences of age. Although this is in part due to the decreased numbers, other statistical procedures such as multiple regression analysis showed that hormone level accounted for only a very minor portion of the behavioural variance, while a much larger percentage was accounted for by age. The various age groups were broken down into tertiles according to whether the free T or LH was high, medium or low. Subsequent two-way analysis of variance showed a significant effect of age on libido and performance but no effect of free T; LH had a significant effect ($P < 0.02$) on performance but not on libido (Table 2).

As in all gerontological research, the confounding factor of disease has to be dealt with. In two recent studies no significant decline in total or free T

Table 1. Spearman rank correlation coefficients between hormones and behaviour in 220 men aged 41 to 93. Only significant correlations are shown. See text for further details (From Davidson et al, unpublished data 1982)

	Libido			Performance						
	Gen. Score+	Feels	Drive	Gen. Score+	Org. Frequ.	Noct. Erect.	Spont. Erect.	Get Erect.	Hold Erect.	Ejac. Capac.
Free T	—	0.13*	—	0.15*	0.19**	—	—	—	—	0.16*
Total T	—	—	—	—	—	—	—	—	—	—
LH	−0.14*	—	—	−0.29**	−0.25**	−0.27**	−0.18**	−0.18**	−0.13*	—
FT/E++	0.14*	0.14*	—	0.22**	0.18**	—	0.15*	0.22**	0.20**	0.20**

*$P < 0.05$
**$P < 0.005$
+ Gen. Score: general libido or performance scores for each man were constructed by averaging responses to two libido and six performance questions, respectively.
++ FT/E: Free T divided by œstradiol.

levels were found in groups of aging men highly selected for physical and mental health and intellectual/educational level (Harman and Tsitouras, 1980; Sparrow, Bosse and Rowe, 1980). The claim was made that in the many other studies in which a T decline was found this effect was due to ill health (Harman and Tsitouras, 1980). This has not, however, been substantiated, and in our study multiple regression analysis failed to show that disease (or alcohol consumption) were major factors in determining T level. Likewise, Tsitouras, Martin and Harman (1982) found that exceptionally healthy men showed a significant decline in sexual activity (50 per cent decrease, based on retrospective interview data) from early sixties to late seventies.

Table 2. *Sexual performance (rated 1 to 5), a composite score of frequency of sexual activities and degree of potency in men grouped by age and by tertiles of free T index or LH. Tertile limits were based on approximate mean values for youngest and oldest age groups. Two-way analysis of variance: Age, $P < 0.001$; free T, $P > 0.05$; LH, $P < 0.03$. (From Davidson et al, unpublished data 1982)*

	Free testosterone (pg/ml)			Luteinizing hormone (ng/ml)		
	< 120	120—180	> 180	< 60	60—110	> 110
40—49	4.5	3.9	3.7	3.9	3.8	4.7
50—59	3.3	3.5	4.0	3.8	3.9	3.1
60—69	3.5	3.2	3.2	3.6	3.0	3.0
70—93	2.2	2.3	3.0	3.1	2.2	2.3

The concept of male climacteric, involving precipitous decline in T and associated menopause-like symptoms, is accepted in some clinical circles (Van Keep, Serr and Greenblatt, 1979). If it exists as a defined clinical entity, however, it is probably extremely rare (admittedly no large-scale surveys have yet been conducted). Thus frank hypogonadism may be almost as rare in the aging population as among younger adults, and the aging decrease in androgen is apparently not sufficient to have a major impact on sexuality. It remains possible, however, that sexual decline represents a quite variable change in androgen sensitivity of the behavioural target tissues (wherever they are!), so that the severity of this defect (in receptors?) is not correlated well with the level of free or total T. The fact that there is a somewhat better relationship to LH is consistent with this idea. LH increase signifies the response of hypothalamic-pituitary tissue to lowered androgen and *might* therefore reflect a shift in CNS androgen receptor sensitivity which is also relevant to behaviour change (see Davidson, Gray and Smith, 1981).

Tsitouras, Martin and Harman (1982) have recently observed that when 183 men aged 60 to 79 were grouped in tertiles according to (remembered) level of sexual activity during the previous year, the group with highest activity had a slightly but significantly higher total T level than the others. Since this population of men, highly selected for good health, was previously found not to show an overall, significant age-related decline in total or free T (Harman and Tsitouras, 1980) and the behaviour-related T changes were within the normal range, this finding could be interpreted as indicating a receptor or other sensitivity deficit, manifesting in a behavioural effect even when androgen titre was only marginally reduced.

Our conclusions regarding aging are that the vast majority of men with age-related sexual decline are not suffering primarily from androgen deficiency, and that it remains to be demonstrated that T treatment is truly efficacious in any but the rare aging individuals who have extremely low circulating T (see the section after next). Nevertheless, further research is required to examine the possibility that decreased sensitivity to the behavioural effects of androgen plays a significant role in sexual deficits of the aged man.

ANDROGEN REPLACEMENT FOR HYPOSEXUALITY IN HYPOGONADAL MEN

There are many clinical reports on androgen replacement which mention effects on sexual behaviour or experience (see e.g., Money, 1961), but usually only *en passant* and invariably without controls and/or reliable, detailed assessment of the elements of sexual function. In 1979 Davidson, Camargo and Smith published a double-blind, placebo (DBP) crossover study assessing the effects of monthly injections of 100 or 400 mg of T enanthate in six hypogonadal men. Each subject kept detailed daily logs of sexual function throughout the 4 to 6 months of the study. The total frequency of erections, from any form of sexual activity or 'spontaneous', consistently increased and decreased within a week or so following the respective rise and fall of plasma T level (Figure 2). In addition to the 'total erections' measure, coital and nocturnal erection frequencies showed statistically significant increments. Masturbation and orgasm frequencies manifested clearly positive trends with treatment, but the small number and large variability precluded statistical significance.

With a similar type of experimental design, Skakkebaek et al (1980) studied 12 hypogonadal men (six hypogonadotrophic and six hypergonadotrophic). Oral T undecanoate (160 mg daily) and placebo were compared and significant increases were found in frequency of sexual thoughts, with and without accompanying excitement, and in frequency of ejaculation, both recorded in daily diaries. They also noted a decrease in 'problems with erections', as assessed by interview ratings.

Luisi and Franchi (1980), in a shorter double-blind study of orally-active androgens, also used daily assessments to compare the effects of four weeks' administration to primary hypogonadal patients of either T undecanoate (120 mg/d, n = 12) or mesterolone (150 mg/d, n = 14). There was a decline in sexual function in the subjects during three weeks of withdrawal from their routine replacement therapy with injected preparations of T. Significant stimulation by T of libido and of erections and ejaculations during intercourse was obtained when results were compared with pretreatment levels, while an upward trend for mesterolone was not statistically significant (Figure 3). No details on hormone levels were represented, and mesterolone-treated group showed slightly higher responses than the

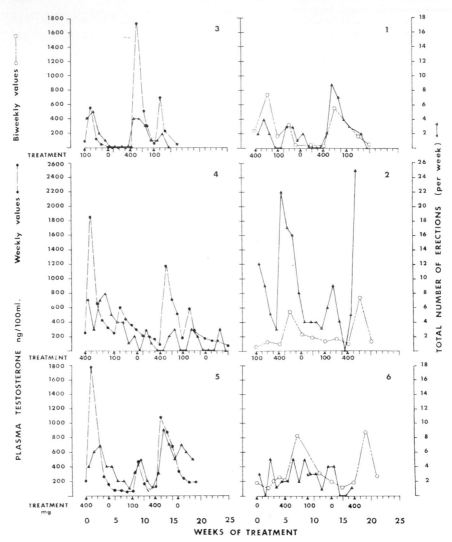

Figure 2. Total erections (however elicited), summated for each week and recorded at the mid-point of the week, for six hypogonadal men, in relation to testosterone enanthate treatment and plasma T level. Individual plasma T presented weekly (subjects 3 to 5) or bi-weekly (subjects 1, 2 and 6). From Davidson, Camargo and Smith (1979).

T-treated one on all measures before treatment. All subjects presumably knew they were receiving an androgen and the placebo-alone condition was not used. Nevertheless, strong placebo effects are not generally found in androgen replacement experiments.

In a final DBP study Lunglmayr, Stellamor and Spona (1980) gave 75 mg of mesterolone per day to 17 impotent men aged 45 to 65, selected according to whether they had a certain minimum out of a total of 31 psychological and somatic symptoms said to characterize the 'male climacteric'. They

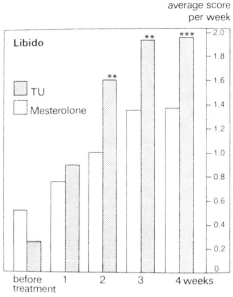

- Average weekly scores of libido. Statistically significant difference as compared with M: ** p < 0.01 *** p < 0.001.

Figure 3. Effects of the orally administered androgens testosterone undecanoate (TU) and mesterolone on libido, assessed daily on a scale of 0 to 4. From Luisi and Franchi (1980).

concluded that mesterolone did improve potency in these men, but the statistical analysis showed a P value of 0.1. Other reasons why this study is essentially not interpretable include the superficial presentation of behavioural data and the lack of information as to how many of the subjects were truly hypogonadal and what their responses were.

It has been claimed that androgen replacement therapy is less effective sexually in hypogonadotrophic than in hypergonadotrophic hypogonadal patients (Money and Clopper, 1975; Money and Dalery, 1977). While this is true for somatic effects, it has not been substantiated experimentally for sexual behaviour, and no difference was noted in the DBP study of Skakkebaek et al (1980) between the two classes of hypogonadal men.

Missing in all studies to date has been any systematic assessment of the 'libidinous' elements of pleasure, satisfaction, or more simply, sensation (in either sense of the word!). Later we shall consider the possibility that, by omitting to study these variables, previous investigators (including ourselves) have to an extent 'missed the boat' as far as understanding the essential role of androgen in sexuality is concerned.

DOSE-RESPONSE RELATIONSHIPS AND THEIR LATENCIES

Two types of information are required in order to establish dose-response curves: (a) the relationships between dose levels and resulting blood levels for specified androgen preparations and routes of administration, and (b) the blood levels of androgen required to restore or maintain any specific level of sexual function. A reasonable amount of data are available on (a), but very little quantitative data from controlled studies are available for definitive conclusions regarding (b). If one takes the normal daily T secretion rate of 5 to 10 mg into account, injections of 100 to 200 mg of a long-acting androgen once each three weeks would supply enough T to bring the hypogonadal patient into that range, given constant release from site of injection and the assumption that distribution, binding and metabolism of T from the injected depot is similar to that secreted by the testes. However, most of this dose will be released in the first week or two since these treatments result in an initial peak followed by a low trough before the next injection (see Figure 4). We need to learn about the effects of these wild swings versus more constant levels both in terms of the therapeutic response and such undesirable side effects as prostate growth.

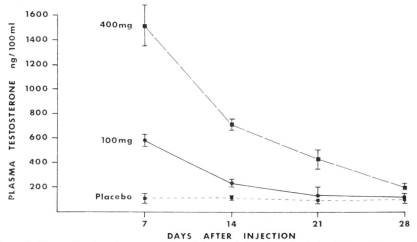

Figure 4. Plasma T values (means ± SE) at different times after injection of 100 or 400 mg of T enanthate in hypogonadal males. From Davidson, Camargo and Smith (1979). See also Sokol et al (1982).

In rats, a constant level of plasma T (generated from Silastic capsules implanted in castrates), which was well below the normal mean, was sufficient to maintain mating behaviour (Damassa, Smith and Davidson, 1977). The normal secretion of T, in both animals and men, is episodic, and the suggestion arising from this study was that exposure to constant T levels is more 'efficient' (i.e., lower mean androgen levels are needed) than is the case with a fluctuating source, i.e., the normal testes. This finding is relevant to establishing appropriate dose levels with subcutaneously implanted T pellets or improved similar slow-release methods of administering free T to men being studied (Marberger, 1976; Frick et al, 1981). It is still undetermined, in any species, whether there are biological advantages to the episodic mode of T release. Pulsatile release is a necessary condition of continued activity of the neuropeptide, LH-releasing hormone (Crowley and McArthur, 1980; Knobil, 1980).

A few data are available which indicate a dose-response relationship using injections of 0, 100 and 400 mg T enanthate (Davidson, Camargo and Smith, 1979). From the same study it was clear that monthly treatment with T enanthate is likely to result in periods of reduced sexuality, and androgen level sinks in the last week or so to hypogonadal levels, with concomitant effects on sexual activity. Since in the above-mentioned study the response to different doses were summed over each four-week injection period, Bancroft (1980) has suggested that these differences might reflect only the more rapid clearance of the lower dose from circulation, and not a true dose-response relationship. Accordingly, we have recalculated the data. Table 3 shows results from the first two weeks of the treatment periods; a significant difference is apparent in total erections from all causes between the two dose levels and each versus placebo.

Table 3. *Total number of sexual events involving erection (including spontaneous erections) in the first two weeks after treatment with T enanthate. Statistical analysis: Friedman analysis of variance followed by Wilcoxon signed ranks test. From data of J. M. Davidson, C. A. Camargo and E. R. Smith*

Subject	Treatment		
	Placebo	100 mg	400 mg
1	0	4	8
2	2	3	6
3	2	8	10
4	9	11	39
5	6	8	10
6	3	6	7
Mean ± S.E.	3.7 ± 1.2	6.7 ± 1.1	13.3 ± 5.2

P value (one tailed): < 0.02 for 100 mg vs. placebo and 400 mg vs 100 mg.

At the present time it seems that the manufacturer's recommended dose range for T enanthate of 200 to 400 mg is appropriate in the light of present knowledge. However, it is preferable to dose at least every three weeks rather than monthly in order to maintain constancy of therapeutic effect (Davidson, Camargo and Smith, 1979), and more often when 1 to 200 mg doses are used (Sokol et al, 1982). The two double-blind studies which reported positive results with the non-hepatotoxic, orally-active T undecanoate used three doses per day of 40 mg (Luisi and Franchi, 1980) and two doses of 80 mg (Skakkebaek et al, 1980) respectively. In the latter study low plasma levels of T were found four hours after oral administration. It appears that this ester is rapidly absorbed and cleared, so that effective doses cannot be achieved without high transient peaks in blood T (see also Geere et al, 1980).

That T undecanoate can stimulate sexual behaviour without raising plasma T levels into the normal range for any length of time (Skakkebaek et al, 1980) raises the interesting question of whether the dose-response curve extends through the rather broad normal range. Expressed differently, does it matter whether a man has a plasma level of 3 or 11 ng/ml? The relationship between levels of T and of sexual function in populations of apparently normal individuals has been addressed in both animals and men. Brown, Monti and Corriveau (1978) found no significant relationship, in 101 young men, between plasma T and frequency of sexual thoughts and orgasm. Kraemer et al (1976) and Raboch and Starka (1973) previously failed to find positive correlations in smaller samples of young adult men. Damassa, Smith and Davidson (1977) found no correlation with the various measures of rat copulatory behaviour, and Harding and Feder (1976) reached a similar conclusion for guinea pigs. This suggests that the effective range of the dose-response curve is below that normally found among healthy young individual mammals, an interpretation experimentally corroborated for rats (Damassa, Smith and Davidson, 1977).

However, the plasma androgen level required to prevent impotence is presumably less than that needed to produce maximal (or optimal) levels of sexuality, and the above-mentioned studies probably would not have detected subtle changes. That T levels within the normal range may influence some aspects of sexual function is indicated by recent results using penile plethysmography, which show a significant positive correlation between latency to full erection (Rubin et al, 1979; Lange et al, 1980) and/or magnitude of erection (Rubin et al, 1979) in response to erotic film on the one hand and plasma T titre on the other. Further research is needed to clarify (a) whether these preliminary data indicate a causal hormone-behaviour relationship; and (b) whether the effect is sufficient to influence significantly a man's sexuality.

The clinical criterion for hypoandrogenicity is generally taken as a plasma T level of < 3 ng/ml. In a single-blind study, described in Chapter 2, Pirke and Kockott provide the only available experimental data on the lower threshold of plasma T required to maintain sexual function in men. Kockott concludes tentatively that the lower threshold for sexual behaviour may vary among individuals within the range of blood levels of 2 to 4.5 ng/ml. There is a need for these initial findings to be substantiated in larger-scale studies and on men with lower levels of sexual function before treatment.

As suggested earlier, a rising androgen threshold with considerable inter-individual difference might explain why some aging men show a sexual decline despite low-normal T levels. We have, accordingly, performed double-blind experiments with T enanthate and placebo on four impotent men (aged 48, 64, 67 and 77), with low or negative nocturnal penile tumescence NPT tests, and low but *not* subclinical levels of T. Each of these men showed improvement in the NPT with T treatment and some form of improvement in sexuality. However, neither of these parameters were restored to normal levels, and psychophysiological tests (plethysmographic response to erotic film and fantasy) remained negative. We have noted, incidentally, that NPT reflects the action of androgen-altering treatments better than psychophysiologic testing in two other patient populations: severely androgen-deficient men receiving T and female-to-male trans-sexuals receiving oestrogen.

Regarding the latency from androgen replacement treatment to effect: clearly T administration does not immediately reinstate sexual function.

However, the studies of Skakkebaek et al (1980) and Davidson, Camargo and Smith (1979) do indicate rather short latency effects on behaviour after both replacement and withdrawal of T (from a few days to two weeks). The earliest response to institution of androgen treatment was a trend noted by Skakkebaek et al (1980) towards increased frequency of sexual thoughts and excitement within the first week of androgen replacement. Effects on sexual activity were obtained in the second week in both studies. Luisi and Franchi (1980) noted significant improvement in libido only in the second week (Figure 3) and in erection and ejaculation in the third, but increasing trends in all three parameters were clearly present one week earlier. In both studies, mood elevation accompanied the sexual changes; Luisi and Franchi (1980) showed a significant improvement of 'mental state' on the *second* week. The variability in socio-psycho-sexual circumstances of men during daily life in the community and the rarity of suitable hypogonadal men make it difficult to obtain reliable data of this kind. However, further studies are certainly indicated on latencies to changing physiological sexual response as well as other parameters of sexuality. In light of the large inter- and intraindividual variability these studies will have to be on a fairly large scale to yield convincing results.

The finding that sexual function responds surprisingly rapidly (within days or weeks) to change in T level seems contradictory to the reports of prolonged retention of sexual function after castration. The nature and possible resolution of this apparent paradox will be discussed in the final section.

DIFFERENTIAL EFFECTS OF DIFFERENT ANDROGENS

The long-standing goal in endocrine pharmacology of developing synthetic androgens, in which the 'androgenic' (reproductive-sexual) actions of the molecule are clearly separated from the metabolic (particularly protein-anabolic) effects, has never been satisfactorily realized (Wilson and Griffin, 1980). Yet the apparently even more demanding aim of separating behavioural from somatic-androgenic effects of androgen is possible at least in animals and, if achievable in humans, could have important applications. This would permit, for instance, specific treatment of hypo-sexuality in men with prostatic cancer, or treatment of women in general while avoiding virilization. Conversely, the development of androgens which virilize but do not stimulate sexual function would be useful for certain other classes of patients such as transsexuals or others for whom a strong virilizing effect is all that is desired

That the achievement of this latter kind of separation is not unrealistic is indicated by the fact that dihydrotestosterone (DHT) has all the classic effects of androgen in rats and some other mammalian species, except for the stimulation of sexual behaviour. In these species, most non-aromatizable androgens tested have been found quite ineffective in the stimulation of male sexual behaviour (for an apparent exception see Yahr and Gerling, 1978), which has given rise to the theory that the behavioural actions of androgen are mediated by aromatization to oestrogen in these species (reviewed by MacLusky and Naftolin, 1981). However, DHT is as effective as T on sexual behaviour in guinea pigs and rhesus monkeys. An attempt has been made to explain the differential effectiveness of DHT in terms of its differential conversion to androstanediol in different species (Gay, 1975, 1976).

Although in humans androgen-dependent tissues differ as to their requirement for 5α-reduction (Bardin and Catterall, 1981), as yet there is no published information on the effects of DHT on human sexuality. This is a matter of potential clinical importance, since it would be desirable to treat with DHT in cases where there is a strong tendency to gynaecomastia or other feminizing effects from aromatization.

In a preliminary inquiry Bancroft, Wu and Davidson (1980, unpublished data) investigated the administration of DHT (20 or 50 mg/day by suppository) in one castrate and two hypogonadal men. Effects on sexuality, if any, were minimal, but this dose was not intended (and did not) raise the DHT level in the blood up to that of the normal range of T in eugonadal men. Treatment with mesterolone, which is also non-aromatizable (Breuer and Gutgemann, 1966), resulted only in statistically insignificant trends in the DBP study of Luisi and Franchi (1980, see Figure 4) and in the less convincing study (see above) of Lunglmayr, Stellamor and Spona (1980). Fluoxymesterone, another non-aromatizable androgen widely used in men, is relatively ineffective in rats (Beach and Westbrook, 1968) and reportedly in men (Reilly and Gordon, 1961) though no controlled study is available. There do not seem to be any controlled studies of its effects on sexual function.

On the other hand, a very brief report by Gooren (1982) indicates a positive effect of DHT. These authors studied six 'agonadal' men who had 'lost testicular function' when they were 16 to 42 years of age. Their ongoing oral T undecanoate treatment (120 mg/d) was substituted with DHT undecanoate in the same dosage for a period of 12 weeks. No deterioration of sexual function was observed during the period of DHT substitution. Further evidence was obtained by administering the anti-oestrogen tamoxifen to 80 infertile men. The dosage was physiologically effective in that increases in FSH, LH, T and oestradiol were observed, but no effects on sexual function were noted even after 12 months of administration. If, as assumed, the tamoxifen was preventing intracellular aromatization by the relevant target tissues for sexual function, these data along with Gooren's DHT experiment strongly suggest that aromatization is not necessary for androgen's sexual function in men. However, extremely sketchy information was supplied on the behavioural observations; thus the question will remain moot until a more thorough presentation of the data and experimental methodology is available.

It remains important that further adequate research be done on the relationship between molecular structure and sexual function of androgens in humans, both for the practical reasons discussed above and in order to clarify the question of what molecular transformations androgen might undergo prior to its action on sexuality.

BEHAVIOURAL MECHANISM OF ACTION OF ANDROGEN

No clinician or researcher who has observed a hypogonadal patient begin his transformation from a eunuchoid state to renewed sexuality at the touch of a needle containing T can fail to experience considerable wonder over how the hormone works. Yet the need to understand the mechanism of the action of androgen on sexual behaviour goes beyond mere curiosity; it is an issue of central importance, not only clinically but also scientifically, since it concerns probably the most phylogenetically stable, biologically important known action of a hormone on behaviour.

The accumulation of past clinical experience and recent controlled studies indicate the likelihood that androgen administration can lead to stimulation of all major elements of sexuality in the hypogonadal man: libido, frequency of sexual activity, erectile potency and ejaculatory capacity, and presumably pelvic and other extragenital sexual response. Are we then to assume that androgen acts directly on all these elements of sexuality? Such a multiple-target arrangement would be unparsimonious, and difficult to investigate. Conversely, is it likely that one primary site of action underlies all these effects? As mentioned above, potency and libido are not independent of each other. Their interactions do not merely manifest in special cases, but are an integral part of the normal sexual response. There is reason to postulate a positive feedback mechanism involving sensory afferents which report genital vasocongestive responses to the brain, thereby increasing sexual arousal which in turn augments physiological responses, leading to the rapid buildup of both cognitive sexual excitement and physiological arousal (Campbell, 1976; Davidson, 1980). If this is so, it may be difficult in a normally-functioning individual (i.e., one with intact sensorimotor mechanisms and libido) to distinguish whether a given variable influences sexual function by acting on libido or potency elements. Analysis of the causal chains involved will undoubtedly require the study of subjects with defined neural, vascular or hormonal defects. But what can we conclude from existing data?

We have previously referred to the apparent inconsistency between long-term retention of sexual activity in a significant percentage of castrates and the recent experimental data indicating rapid effects of androgen withdrawal and replacement on sexual activity involving erections. We suspect that finding the solution to this apparent paradox could greatly contribute to understanding the role of androgen in male sexuality. In virtually the first serious attempt to explain the behavioural effect of androgen in men, Bancroft (1980) presented a novel idea which addresses the issue of the proximate effect of androgen, while also helping us towards a resolution of this paradox. Since withdrawal and replacement of T in hypogonadal men was associated with a waning and waxing of sexual thoughts, and since these changes in sexual thoughts (with or without associated 'excitement') preceded effects on erectile problems and ejaculation (Skakkebaek et al, 1980), he proposed that the effects on erectile potency are mediated strictly by increased 'sexual appetite' (libido), as well as a separate effect on ejaculation. More striking evidence for excluding a direct effect of androgen on erection comes from a laboratory study of Bancroft and Wu (1982) in which two castrates and six hypogonadal men showed erectile responses to erotic film not significantly different from those of normal controls, or from their own responses during androgen treatment. However, the response to sexual fantasy was suppressed in the untreated condition and was restored by T. The idea that androgen is needed for the response to fantasy but not to film is partly supported by previous work (Bancroft et al, 1974) showing that cyproterone acetate and oestrogen treatment of sex offenders decreased their response to fantasy more than to film: that is, if these agents 'work' only via decreasing T levels, an issue which is still controversial (Laschet, 1973; Freund, 1980).

Bancroft concludes that (apart from its role in ejaculation) androgen acts on sexuality via cognitive acts involved in generation of sexual imagery, specifically improved maintenance of attention. He garners support for this view from research on chickens indicating increased persistence of food searching behaviour in T-treated birds (Andrew, 1972). Bancroft compares this effect with statements by hypogonadal men who have trouble concentrating on thoughts of sex or 'general intellectual tasks'. He describes this putative androgen-dependent function as an active cognitive process and suggests that it may be responsible for the well-known sex difference in visuo-spatial ability.

The idea that T affects erection largely by effects on libido helps to solve the above-mentioned paradox because it implies that castrates need not lose the capacity for erection, or at least not for a long time post-operatively. Although not motivated to have erections, they could conceivably generate them in order to satisfy their sexual partner.

It is hard to evaluate Bancroft's analogy with androgenic facilitation of persistence in chickens, since the behaviour is so far removed from that of sexual fantasy in men. Though the influence of T on persistence has been extended to mice by Archer (1977) and rats by Thompson and Wright (1979) the interpretation of the behavioural effects is by no means clear, as the latter authors point out. Moreover, this action of T is pharmacological, at least in the studies on mammals, since T levels were raised far above the normal range. The only relevant studies on T and cognitive functions in men (Broverman, Klaiber and Vogel, 1980) found that high androgen level facilitated performance on stereotyped repetitive tasks such as serial subtraction (i.e., it was conducive to 'automatization' of behaviour). This effect is consistent with the animal findings, though less likely with the active process of generation and maintenance of imagery in men.

In this laboratory we have been able to confirm, in two castrates and one man with a plasma T of < 1 ng/ml, that film-induced changes in penile circumference were at least as large as, if not larger than, those of normal controls, and were unchanged by T replacement. However, unlike Bancroft's findings, responses during fantasy were robust and unaffected by androgen deficiency or its replacement. Furthermore, our subjects failed to show the rapid detumescence found in normal volunteers after termination of the three- or four-minute film or fantasy episodes, even when cognitive effort (e.g., mental arithmetic) was used in the attempt to distract the subject from possibly arousing attention to sexual thoughts. We surmise that the difference between the response of Bancroft's subjects to film and fantasy has to do with quantitative differences between the arousing properties of the two kinds of stimulus, a possibility also admitted by Bancroft (1980). However, we cannot explain the difference between his (Scottish) subjects and our (Californian) ones, though both series (especially ours) are small and more subjects will have to be studied to determine which pattern is more general.

Is there more evidence that, contrary to widespread medical belief and animal experience (Davidson et al, 1978), T is not necessary for erection? As mentioned above, Eibl (1978) is reported to have observed 'full erection' in response to film in an appreciable percentage of castrated sex offenders, three to five years after castration, though we have no further information on this study. There is also support for Bancroft's finding that libido is affected before erectile potency in the data of Luisi and Franchi (1980). Yet we are faced with the apparently inconsistent observations that hypo-gonadal and castrate men report severe problems of sexual dysfunction, decrease or cease sexual activity, and often refer their perceived deficiencies in sexual capacity to problems with erection. These deficiencies are reduced or abolished with T treatment. One suspects that some aspects(s) of erectile potency which are not measured in the laboratory studies are affected by androgen. What might this be? Since these patients often report that their difficulties in intercourse are related to inability to *maintain* erection, is it that the laboratory situation misleads by measuring only short periods of exposure to arousing stimuli? If so, however, one would expect rapid detu-mescence when or before the stimulus is removed, and what we have encountered in the laboratory is prolonged maintenance of erection after the film or fantasy is terminated. Is it simply a question of rigidity, since some investigators believe that full circumference increases may be present without final achievement of sufficient rigidity for normal intromission (Karacan, 1982)? It is, however, still not established that this phenomenon is a frequent cause of sexual failure, though is may occur in rare patho-logical defects of the penile vasculature. At any rate we tested the rigidity of the erection of a castrate off replacement therapy (plasma T in hypogonadal range for about one month) and found that it resisted buckling at pressures in excess of 1000 g (criterion of adequate rigidity = 450 g, Karacan, 1982).

What we suspect may be a major factor is a vital aspect of sexuality not generally assessed in sex research and not mentioned in the studies discussed above: the enjoyment of sexual activity or, more specifically, *pleasurable awareness of sexual response*. This is not unrelated to Bancroft's notion of sexual 'appetite' as mediator of androgen action, since both desire and pleasure are elements which belong in the category of libido. The difference is that his concept of appetite is tied to the cerebral cognitive activity involved in fantasy, while ours has to do at least in part with sensory function, involving effects of androgen on genital sensory receptors or afferent pathways to the CNS instead of, or in addition to, action on the brain. The simplest model would involve a direct effect of T to lower the threshold of genital sensation in receptors whose activation stimulates sexual desire as well as erection. But wherever the site(s) of this putative action of androgen are, the emphasis on sensory hedonic systems stands in contrast to the hypothesis that the cognitive generation and maintenance of imagery is primary for androgen action.

Biological support for the proposal that sensory afferents may play a role in erection can be found in animal research. In rats spontaneous erections, which occur rhythmically when rats are held supine with the prepuce retracted and without tactile stimuli, are inhibited by penile deafferentation (Sachs and Garinello, 1980) or local anaesthesia (Stefanick and Davidson, 1982). This indicates a role of sensory afferents in the rhythmic cycle of erections which is mediated by spinal reflex action (Hart, 1967). Likewise in men, initial tumescence from whatever stimulus could facilitate full erection by means of activating sensory afferents which also generate pleasure reactions, especially in the presence of a sexual context.

In further attempting to explain the surprisingly slow detumescence of our castrate/hypogonadal subjects, we tentatively suggest that the same sensory input from the genitals involved in initiation of erection may be involved in its termination (without orgasm). This may in fact be the source of information, in the normally androgenized male, necessary to couple erectile responses to onset/offset of sexual stimuli. Thus, in the absence of this modulating influence of T, erection is maintained even when the stimulus is switched off. A criticism of this suggestion might be that younger men maintain erections longer than older ones (and they are sexually more vigorous and have higher T levels). But this may have nothing to do with androgen, but rather with such factors as non-endocrine-dependent deterioration of sensory receptors consequent to aging (Newman, 1970; Edwards and Husted, 1976). We propose therefore that the castrate's erections may be both uncontrolled and lacking in pleasurable genital sensations.

The proposed hypothesis implies that androgen acts to facilitate sensitivity to or pleasurable awareness of *both* sexual thoughts and activity, since both involve the same physiological response. At this point we would not attempt to specify whether the initial 'awareness' is necessarily fully conscious, nor whether the primary event in sexual arousal is the initial physiological process (as suggested by Campbell, 1976) or the thought, since we think the two are linked in a positive feedback relationship. In the absence of T, erections might proceed to completion only if directly driven by strong visual, tactile or cognitive stimuli. Spontaneous erections would tend to be absent in hypogonadism if they depended on the positive feedback influence of pleasurable awareness of sexual response or at least of lowered sensitivity to stimulation. In fact we have found that T stimulated the occurrence of spontaneous erections in each of three castrates. Moreover, oestrogen, in androgen-depleting doses, reduced them in each of six male-to-female pre-surgical transsexuals, when treated in a DBP experiment, though their (mostly robust) erectile responses to fantasy and film were not significantly affected by the hormone treatments (Kwan and Davidson, 1982 unpublished data). Interestingly, sleep-related spontaneous erections are also affected by androgen. Thus, directly measured NPT responses were significantly increased by T in five out of five of the above-mentioned transsexuals. Previously, self-reported nocturnal erections were found to increase significantly with T treatment in hypogonadal men (Davidson, Camargo and Smith, 1979). This was recently corroborated by direct measurement in two castrates and one severely hypogonadal man, and it suggests that some analogue of the waking pleasurable awareness of spontaneous erections or at least of genital sensitivity still operates in sleep, though not necessarily manifesting itself in dream content.

The behaviour-reinforcing properties of sexual pleasure could suffice to explain all effects of androgen on sexuality through a 'domino' process involving increased sexual thoughts or fantasies, spontaneous erections (including nocturnal ones), coitus or masturbation, satisfaction and even ejaculation. As for the last-mentioned element, Bancroft (1980) has proposed a direct effect of androgen thereupon. There are still no data to support an action of androgen directly on any aspect of the orgasmic/ejaculatory process other than the production of semen by the accessory glands, and seminal emission is clearly not essential for orgasm (Beach, Westbrook and Clemens, 1966; Davidson, 1980). Thus it seems to us more likely that hypogonadal men are anorgasmic because they fail to reach the level of sexual arousal required to trigger the orgasmic response than for lack of semen. Genital afferents surely carry much of the sensory information involved in this build-up of arousal until some orgasmic threshold is reached (Masters and Johnson, 1966; Sherfey, 1972; Davidson, 1980; for animal model, see Bermant and Davidson, 1974, p. 111). It is consistent with our hypothesis and existing data to propose that androgen is involved in a facilitation of sensation/pleasurable awareness originating in this process, which in turn contributes both to the occurrence and intensity of orgasm.

SUMMARY

Only in the last few years has the scientific study of hormonal replacement therapy for hyposexuality begun in earnest with the advent of appropriately controlled experimental studies. Dose-response relationships can be demonstrated between testosterone (T) and sexual measures, but these have not yet been investigated in detail. Some aspects of sexual function are maintained in the presence of androgen levels well below the normal range, but preliminary evidence suggests that within a normal population high levels of T are correlated with more vigorous responses to visual erotic stimuli. Though T (and to a greater extent free T) declines with aging in parallel with the decline of sexual function, these hormonal changes contribute only to a minor extent to the behavioural change. Some non-aromatizable androgens may be less effective in stimulating sexual behaviour than T, but initial data on effects of dihydrotestosterone suggests that the capacity of an androgen to be aromatized (converted to oestrogen) is not a requirement for its sexual action. While T apparently increases the incidence of all types of male sexual activity, recent data contradict the belief that it directly facilitates the erectile mechanism in men, even though erection frequency is greatly reduced in untreated hypogonadal men. At the present juncture, it appears that the initial action of T may be on libido factors which lead in turn to the stimulation of other aspects of sexuality. Specifically, we propose that androgen acts through stimulating genital sensations and/or other pleasurable awareness of sexual response rather than directly through cognitive processes such as sexual imagery.

ACKNOWLEDGEMENTS

This work was supported by National Institutes of Health Grant AG 1437.

REFERENCES

Andrew, R. J. (1972) Changes in search behavior in male and female chicks, following different doses of testosterone. *Animal Behavior,* **20,** 741-750.

Archer, J. (1977) Testosterone and persistence in mice. *Animal Behavior,* **25,** 479-488.

Bancroft, J. (1980) Endocrinology of sexual function. *Clinics in Obstetrics and Gynaecology,* **7,** 253-281.

Bancroft, J. & Wu, F. C. W. (1982) Changes in erectile responsiveness during androgen replacement therapy. *Archives of Sexual Behavior* (in press).

Bancroft, J., Tennent, T. G., Loucas, K. & Cass, J. (1974) Control of deviant sexual behavior by drugs: behavioural effects of oestrogens and anti-androgens. *British Journal of Psychiatry,* **125,** 310-315.

Baker, H. W. G., Burger, H. G., deKretser, D. M., Hudson, B., O'Connor, S., Wang, C., Mirovics, A., Court, J., Dunlop, M. & Rennie, G. C. (1976) Changes in the pituitary-testicular system with age. *Clinical Endocrinology,* **5,** 349-372.

Bardin, C. W. & Catterall, J. F. (1981) Testosterone: a major determinant of extragenital sexual dimorphism. *Science,* **211,** 1285-1293.

Beach, F. A. (1948) *Hormones and Behavior.* New York: Hoeber.

Beach, F. A., Westbrook, W. H. & Clemens, L. G. (1966) Comparisons of the ejaculatory responses — men and animals. *Psychosomatic Medicine,* **28,** 749-763.

Beach, G. A. & Westbrook, W. H. (1968) Dissociation of androgenic effects on sexual morphology and behavior in male rats. *Endocrinology,* **83,** 395-398.

Bermant, G. & Davidson, J. M. (1974) *Biological Bases of Sexual Behavior.* New York: Harper and Row.

Breuer, H. & Gutgemann, D. (1966) Wirkung von 1a-methyl-5a-androstan-17β-ol-3-on (mesterolon) auf die steroidausscheidung beim menschen. *Arzneimittel Forschung,* **16,** 759.

Broverman, D. M., Klaiber, E. L. & Vogel, W. (1980) Gonadal hormones and cognitive functioning. In *The Psychobiology of Sex Differences and Sex Roles* (Ed.) Parsons, E. pp. 57-80. Washington: Hemisphere Publishing Co.

Brown, W. A., Monti, P. M. & Corriveau, D. P. (1978) Serum testosterone and sexual activity and interest in men. *Archives of Sexual Behavior,* **7,** 97-103.

Campbell, B. (1976) Neurophysiology of the clitoris. In *The Clitoris*, (Ed.) Lowry, T. P. & Lowry, T. S. pp. 35-73. St. Louis: W. H. Green.

Crowley, W. F. & McArthur, J. W. (1980) Stimulation of the normal menstrual cycle in Kallman's syndrome by pulsatile administration of luteinizing hormone-releasing hormone (LHRH). *Journal of Clinical Endocrinology and Metabolism,* **51,** 173-175.

Damassa, D. A., Smith, E. R. & Davidson, J. M. (1977) The relationship between circulating testosterone levels and sexual behavior. *Hormones and Behavior,* **8,** 275-286.

Davidson, J. M. (1980) The psychobiology of sexual experience. In *The Psychobiology of Consciousness* (Ed.) Davidson, J. M. & Davidson, R. J. pp. 271-332. New York: Plenum Press.

Davidson, J. M., Camargo, C. A. & Smith, E. R. (1979) Effects of androgen on sexual behavior in hypogonadal men. *Journal of Clinical Endocrinology and Metabolism,* **48,** 955-958.

Davidson, J. M., Gray, G. D. & Smith, E. R. (1979) Animal models in the endocrinology of reproductive behavior. In *Animal Models for Research on Contraception and Fertility* (Ed.) Alexander, N. pp. 61-81. Hagerstown, Md.: Harper & Row.

Davidson, J. M., Gray, G. D. & Smith, E. R. (1982) The sexual psychoendocrinology of ageing. In *Neuroendocrinology of Aging* (Ed.) Meites, J. (in press). New York: Plenum Press.

Davidson, J. M., Stefanick, M. L., Sachs, B. L. & Smith, E. R. (1978) Role of androgen in sexual reflexes of the male rat. *Physiology & Behavior,* **21,** 141-146.

Davidson, J. M., Chen, J. J., Crapo, L., Gray, G. D. & Greenleaf, W. J. (1982) Hormonal changes and sexual functions in men (unpublished data).

Edwards, A. E. & Husted, J. R. (1976) Penile sensitivity, age and sexual behavior. *Journal of Clinical Psychology,* **32,** 697-700.

Eibl, E. (1978) Treatment and after-care of 300 sex offenders, especially with regard to penile plethysmography. In *Justizministerium Baden-Wurttemberg* (Ed.), *Proceedings of the German Conference on Treatment Possibilities for Sex Offenders in Eppingen,* 1977, Stuttgart (in German).

Freund, K. (1980) Therapeutic sex drive reduction. *Acta Psychiatrica Scandinavica* (Supplement 62) 5-38.

Frick, J., Bende, T., Aulitzky, H. & Schmidt, F. (1981) Subdermal implants of different steroidal compounds for treatment of endocrinological disorders. *European Urology,* **7,** 73-77.

Gay, V. L. (1975) Ineffectiveness of DHT treatment in producing increased serum DHT in orchidectomized rats: evidence for rapid *in vitro* metabolism of DHT to androstanediol. *Federation Proceedings,* **34,** 303, abstract.

Gay, V. L. (1976) Species variation in the metabolism of dihydrotestosterone: correlation with reported variations in behavioral response. *Abstracts of the 9th Annual Meeting of the Society for the Study of Reproduction,* 1976.

Geere, G., Jones, J., Atherden, S. M. & Grant, D. B. (1980) Plasma androgens after a single oral dose of testosterone undecanoate. *Archives of Diseases in Childhood,* **55.** 218-220.

Gooren, L. (1982) Aromatization of testosterone to estradiol is not required for maintenance of sexual behavior in the male. *Proceedings of the 5th World Congress of Sexology, Jerusalem, 1981* (in press).

Gray, G. D., Smith, E. R., Dorsa, D. M. & Davidson, J. M. (1981) Sexual behavior and testosterone in middle-aged male rats. *Endocrinology,* **109,** 1597-1604.

Harding, C. F. & Feder, H. H. (1976) Relation between individual differences in sexual behavior and plasma testosterone levels in the guinea pig. *Endocrinology,* **98,** 1198-1205.

Harman, S. M. & Tsitouras, P. D. (1980) Reproductive hormones in aging men. I. Measurement of sex steroids, basal luteinizing hormone, and leydig cell response to human chorionic gonadotropin. *Journal of Clinical Endocrinology and Metabolism,* **51,** 35-40.

Hart, B. (1967) Testosterone regulation of sexual reflexes in spinal male rats. *Science,* **155,** 1283-1284.

Heim, N. (1981) Sexual behavior of castrated sex offenders. *Archives of Sexual Behavior,* **10,** 11-19.

Heim, N. & Hursch, C. J. (1979) Castration for sex offenders: treatment or punishment? A review and critique of recent European literature. *Archives of Sexual Behavior,* **8,** 281-305.

Karacan, I. (1982) Evaluation of nocturnal penile tumescence and impotence. In *Sleeping and Waking Disorders: Indications and Techniques* (Ed.) Christian Guilleminault. pp. 343-371. Menlo Park, Ca.: Addison Wesley.

Kinsey, A. C., Pomeroy, W. B. & Martin, C. E. (1948) *Sexual Behavior in the Human Male.* Philadelphia: Saunders.

Kinsey, A. C., Pomeroy, W. B., Martin, C. E. & Gebhard, P. H. (1953) *Sexual Behavior in the Human Female.* Philadelphia: Saunders.

Knobil, E. (1980) The neuroendocrine control of the menstrual cycle. *Recent Progress in Hormone Research,* **36,** 53.

Kraemer, H. C., Becker, H. B., Brodie, H. K. H., Doering, C. H., Moos, R. H. & Hamburg, D. A. (1976) Orgastic frequency and plasma testosterone levels in normal human males. *Archives of Sexual Behavior,* **5,** 125-132.

Lange, J. D., Brown, W. A., Wincze, J. P. & Zwick, W. (1980) Serum testosterone concentration and penile tumescence changes in men. *Hormones and Behavior,* **14,** 267-270.

Laschet, U. (1973) Antiandrogen in the treatment of sex offenders: mode of action and therapeutic outcome. In *Contemporary Sexual Behavior: Critical Issues in the 1970's,* (Ed.) Zubin, J. & Money, J. pp. 311-319. Baltimore: Johns Hopkins University Press.

Luisi, M. & Franchi, F. (1980) Double-blind group comparative study of testosterone undecanoate and mesterolone in hypogonadal male patients. *Journal of Endocrinologic Investigation,* **3,** 305-308.

Lunglmayr, G., Stellamor, M. & Spona, J. (1980) Androgenbehandlung der impotentia coeundi alternder manner. *Wiener Klinische Wochenschrift,* **92,** 243-247.

Maclusky, N. J. & Naftolin, F. (1981) Sexual differentiation of the central nervous system. *Science,* **211,** 1294-1306.

Marberger, L. L. (1976) Hormonal therapy with steroid-filled silastic rubber implants. *British Journal of Urology,* **48,** 153-154.

Masters, W. H. & Johnson, V. E. (1966) *Human Sexual Response.* Boston: Little Brown.

Mitamura, T. (1970) *Chinese Eunuchs.* Tokyo: Charles E. Tuttle.

Money, J. (1961) Sex hormones and other variables in human eroticism. In *Sex and Internal Secretions* (Ed.) Young, W. C. Vol II, Third Edition, pp. 1383-1400. Baltimore, MD: Williams & Wilkins.

Money, J. & Clopper, R. (1975) Postpubertal psychosexual function in post-surgical male hypopituitarism. *Journal of Sex Research,* **11,** 25-38.

Money, J. & Dalery, J. (1977) Sexual disorders: hormonal and drug therapy. In *Handbook of Sexology* (Ed.) Money, J. & Musaph, H. pp. 1303-1310. Amsterdam: Excerpta Medica.

Newman, H. F. (1970) Vibratory sensitivity of the penis. *Fertility and Sterility,* **21,** 791-793.

Raboch, J. & Starka, L. (1973) Reported coital activity of men and levels of plasma testosterone. *Archives of Sexual Behavior,* **2,** 309-315.

Reilly, W. A. & Gordan, G. S. (1961) Dissociation of growth-stimulating and skeleton-maturing actions of the synthetic androgen, fluoxmesterone. *Journal of Pediatrics,* **59,** 188-193.

Rubin, H. B., Henson, D. E., Falvo, R. E. & High, R. W. (1979) The relationship between men's endogenous levels of testosterone and their penile responses to erotic stimuli. *Behavior Research and Therapy,* **17,** 305-312.

Sachs, B. D. & Garinello, L. D. (1980) Hypothetical spinal pacemaker regulating penile reflexes in rats: evidence from transection of spinal cord and dorsal penile nerves. *Journal of Compatative Physiological Psychology,* **94,** 530-535.

Sherfey, M. J. (1972) *The Nature and Evolution of Female Sexuality.* New York: Random House.

Skakkebaek, N. E., Bancroft, L., Davidson, D. W. & Warner, P. (1980) Androgen replacement with oral testosterone undecanoate in hypogonadal men: a double-blind controlled study. *Clinical Endocrinology,* **14,** 49-61.

Sokol, R. Z., Palacios, A., Campfield, L. A., Saul, C. & Swerdloff, R. S. (1982) Comparison of the kinetics of injectable testosterone in eugonadal and hypogonadal men. *Fertility and Sterility,* **37,** 425-430.

Sparrow, D., Bosse, R. & Rowe, J. W. (1980) The influence of age, alcohol consumption, and body build on gonadal function in men. *Journal of Clinical Endocrinology and Metabolism,* **51,** 508-512.

Stearns, E. L., MacDonnel, J. A., Kaufman, B. J., Lucman, T. S., Winter, J. S. & Faiman, C. (1976) Declining testicular function with age. *American Journal of Medicine,* **57,** 761-766.

Stefanick, M. L. & Davidson, J. M. (1982) Suppression of penile reflexes of intact rats following anesthetization of the penis. *Physiology and Behavior* (in press).

Sturup, G. K. (1979) Castration: the total treatment. In *Sexual Behavior: Social and Legal Aspects.* (Ed.) Resnick, H. L. P. & Wolfgang, M. E. pp. 361-382. Boston: Little, Brown.

Thompson, W. R. & Wright, J. S. (1979) 'Persistence' in rats: effects of testosterone. *Physiological Psychology,* **7,** 291-294.

Tsitouras, P. D., Martin, C. E. & Harman, S. M. (1982) Relationship of serum testosterone to sexual activity in healthy elderly men. *Journal of Gerontology,* **37,** 288-293.

Van Keep, P. A., Serr, D. M. & Greenblatt, R. B. (Ed.) (1979) *Female and Male Climacteric.* Baltimore: University Park Press.

Verwoerdt, A., Pfeiffer, E. & Wang, H. S. (1969a) Sexual behavior in senescence — changes in sexual activity and interest of aging men and women. *Journal of Geriatric Psychiatry,* **2,** 163-180.

Verwoerdt, A., Pfeiffer, E. & Wang, H. S. (1969b) Sexual behavior in senescence. *Geriatrics,* **24,** 137-154.

Vermeulen, A., Rubens, R. & Verdonck, L. (1972) Testosterone secretion and metabolism in male senescence. *Journal of Clinical Endocrinology and Metabolism,* **34,** 730-735.

Wasserman, M. D., Pollak, C. P., Spielman, A. J. & Weitzman, E. D. (1980) Theoretical and technical problems in the measurement of nocturnal penile tumescence for the differential diagnosis of impotence. *Psychosomatic Medicine,* **42,** 575-585.

Wilson, J. D. & Griffin, J. E. (1980) The use and misuse of androgens. *Metabolism,* **29,** 1278-1295.

Wolf, C. (1934) *Die Kastration bei sexuellen perversionen und sittlichkeitsverbrechen des mannes.* Basel; B. Schwabe.

Yahr, P. & Gerling, S. A. (1978) Aromatization and androgen stimulation of sexual behavior in male and female rats. *Hormones and Behavior,* **10,** 128-142.

2

Endocrinology of Sexual Dysfunction

K. M. PIRKE
G. KOCKOTT

Sexual dysfunction may develop as a symptom of fatigue resulting from any severe disease, and this non-specific effect may occur in endocrine disorders. There are also specific interactions between endocrine disorder and sexual function as found in diabetes mellitus; these are discussed in Chapter 9. In this article we confine our attention to the direct role of gonadal hormones in sexual dysfunction.

GONADAL HORMONES IN THE FEMALE

In the human female the influence of gonadal hormones for sexual behaviour seems to be less important than in the male. During the menstrual cycle the gonadotrophic hormones, luteinizing hormone (LH) and follicle-stimulating hormone (FSH) as well as the gonadal hormones — the oestrogens, the gestagens and the androgens — undergo considerable variations in their plasma concentration. So far there is apparently no clear relationship between these cyclical hormone changes and female sexual activity (see Chapter 3). The role of hormones in the post-menopausal or oophorectomized woman may be more obvious and these are considered in Chapter 4.

The sexual effects of endocrinopathies such as hyperprolactinaemia, Cushing's syndrome and hypopituitarism are of considerable theoretical interest, but as yet there is virtually no systematically collected evidence to refer to. This also applies to the endocrine status of women with sexual dysfunction. One controlled study of the therapeutic effects of testosterone in female sexual dysfunction has been reported (Carnay, Bancroft and Matthews, 1978), but other studies have failed to replicate the findings (see Chapter 4). At the present time, therefore, we can say very little about the endocrinology of sexual dysfunction in women.

GONADAL HORMONES IN THE MALE

With the human male the situation is different from that in the female in that androgens are unequivocally necessary to maintain sexual desire and sexual activity. These androgens are produced in the Leydig cells of the

Clinics in Endocrinology and Metabolism — Vol. 11, No. 3, November 1982.
0300-595X/82/11.03/625 $03.00 © 1982 W. B. Saunders Company Ltd

testes, and the main compound is testosterone. There is another source of androgens, namely the adrenal gland, which produces several androgenic steroids such as dehydroepiandrosterone, androstenediol, androstenedione, to name only the most important. However, all these compounds are of weak androgenic effect, so that the androgen from the adrenal gland cannot compensate for a loss or severe impairment of testicular function. The importance of androgens for male sexual activity has been proved by three observations:

1. Patients who have been castrated have been studied by Bremer (1959), Langeluddecke (1963) and Cornu (1973). All patients reported a decrease of sexual interest and ability, although sexual potency was not totally lost in all patients.
2. Patients suffering from hypogonadism report a loss of sexual interest and erectile impotence which can easily be reversed by treatment with androgenic drugs (Davidson, Camargo and Smith, 1979; Skakkebaek et al, 1981).
3. Antiandrogenic drugs such as cyproterone acetate are able to suppress sexuality in men (Laschet and Laschet, 1971).

On the following pages we shall describe two recent studies in which our group has examined the role of androgen hormones in male sexual dysfunction.

First Study

In the first study we included patients with erectile impotence and with premature ejaculation. The aim of the study was to contribute to the long-standing controversy over whether patients with mainly psychogenic impotence have a disturbed androgen secretion. Ismail et al (1970) reported significantly decreased testosterone secretion in urine. Legros et al (1973) and Raboch, Mellan and Starka (1973) reported plasma testosterone concentrations which were still in the normal range, but lower than those in undisturbed men. In contrast, Lawrence and Swyer (1974), Comhaire and Vermeulen (1975), and Ansari (1975) found plasma testosterone concentrations which were not different from those of normal men.

We believe that these discrepancies exist for two reasons. First, in the majority of the studies cited the diagnostic criteria describing 'psychogenic impotence' are not well enough defined to allow a comparison between different studies. Secondly, none of the authors have taken into account the intraindividual variability of plasma hormone concentrations, which may well obscure smaller differences between patients and normal controls (Santen and Bardin, 1973; Smith et al, 1974). We have attempted to overcome these shortcomings and have studied three forms of psychogenic impotence: primary and secondary erectile impotence and premature ejaculation. The patients were compared with a normal age-matched group. Ten blood samples were obtained from each subject over a period of three hours. LH, total testosterone, and free (not protein-bound) testosterone — the biologically active fraction of plasma testosterone (Anderson, 1974) — were measured.

Patients

To exclude disturbances of sexual behaviour due to sexual inexperience, no patients younger than 20 years of age were included. Patients had to have lived in a continuous partnership for at least three months. Thus confirmatory information could be obtained from the female partner. Only patients whose sexual disturbance had existed for longer than six months were included.

The diagnosis of psychogenic impotence was made after an extensive medical and psychiatric interview with the patient and his partner. A semi-standardized case history was obtained and a physical examination performed in order to exclude patients with clinical symptoms of hypogonadism and other endocrinological diseases. All patients were in good physical health. Patients with psychiatric diseases, especially psychoses, and drug and alcohol addicts were excluded. There was no evidence of homosexual tendencies in any of the patients. Patients living in a severely disturbed partnership which was about to break up were not included, and patients complaining primarily of decreasing sexual interest were also excluded.

Erectile impotence. The patients selected for the study showed the following symptoms: failure to achieve or maintain erection during attempted coitus with their usual partners; mostly active in masturbation and, if so, capable of erection during masturbation; presence of strong anxiety feelings (determined using psychological testing, Dittmar, Kockott and Nusselt, 1977) and avoidance behaviour toward coital activity.

Using the common division of primary and secondary erectile impotence (Masters and Johnson, 1970), it was established that eight patients aged 21 to 56 years (mean, 28.0 years) belonged to the primary group: they had never experienced normal sexual intercourse. Eight patients, aged 29 to 55 years (mean 37.3 years) suffered from the secondary form: the above-described symptoms had occurred after a period of undisturbed sexual behaviour. The duration of the erectile impotence ranged from six months to more than ten years.

Premature ejaculation. Fifteen patients, aged 23 to 43 years (mean 33.8 years), were classified as having premature ejaculation. Ejaculation occurred in these patients before, at the moment of, or immediately after intromission of the penis. Two subgroups were formed on the basis of whether or not psychological testing (Dittmar, Kockott and Nusselt, 1977) and interview revealed anxiety feelings and avoidance behaviour toward coital activity. Eight patients (group E_2), aged 23 to 43 years (mean 30.2 years), showed anxiety feelings and avoidance behaviour, while the other seven (group E_1), aged 29 to 43 years (mean 38.4), did not show these symptoms.

Normal control subjects

Sixteen subjects, aged 22 to 45 (mean 32.4) years, were classified as normal. They were healthy adult males who, together with their female partners, volunteered for the study. All were in good health, as thorough physical and psychiatric examination revealed. As judged from the information given by the subjects and their partners, their sexual behaviour was undisturbed.

Blood sampling

Between 9 and 10 o'clock in the morning, a needle (butterfly) was inserted into a forearm vein. Ten blood samples of 5 ml each were collected every 20 min. Serum was separated by centrifugation and stored at $-30°C$ until analysed.

LH was measured by radioimmunoassay according to Odell et al (1967). Results were expressed as nanograms of the MRC standard 69-104 per millilitre. Antiserum and LH for iodination were provided by the NIHMD. The intraassay variability was 7.4 per cent at a concentration of 14.7 ng/ml. The average LH concentration was calculated for each subject.

All ten serum samples from each normal subject or patient were pooled and then analysed for testosterone and free testosterone. Testosterone was measured by radioimmunoassay according to Pirke (1973). The interassay variability was 7 per cent at a concentration of 579 ng/100 ml. The free (not protein-bound) testosterone was measured according to Pirke and Doerr (1975). At a concentration of 12.2 ng/100 ml the interassay variability was 9.2 per cent.

Results and discussion

The hormone concentrations in the blood of the patients and of the normal controls are listed in Table 1. For all hormones a Kruskall-Wallis test was performed. No significant differences were found between the groups. The normal ranges as established in our laboratory are indicated on the left side of Table 1.

Evidence has been presented which indicates that sexual activity and sexual stimulation may stimulate the pituitary gonadal system in men. Fox et al (1972) reported elevated androgen secretion after sexual activity. Pirke, Kockott and Dittmar (1974) observed increased plasma testosterone as a response to watching a sexually stimulating film, and Kraemer et al (1976) reported increased plasma testosterone at times of sexual activity in men. Adverse effects of psychogenic stress on the pituitary gonadal system in men were reported by Kreuz, Rose and Jennings (1972), who observed depressed testosterone concentrations in military officer candidates during an especially stressful part of their training.

The data reported here, which are in agreement with the observations of Lawrence and Swyer (1974), Ansari (1975), Comhaire and Vermeulen (1975) and Schwarz, Kolodny and Masters (1980), indicate that androgen deficiency does not contribute to the development of psychogenic erectile impotence and premature ejaculation. On the other hand, decreased plasma testosterone concentrations were reported by Legros et al (1973) and Raboch, Mellan and Starka (1975). It is conceivable that either the reduced sexual activity of the patients or the stressful situation brought about by the patients' fears of sexual failure could explain the observations of the latter two groups. Our data do not support the latter assumption, since the

Table 1. *Hormone concentrations in the blood of patients with sexual disturbance and of normal control subjects*

	Normal range	Primary erectile impotence $\bar{x} \pm SEM^a$	Secondary erectile impotence $\bar{x} \pm SEM^a$	Premature ejaculation		Control group $\bar{x} \pm SEM^a$	P
				group E_1 $\bar{x} \pm SEM^a$	group E_2 $\bar{x} \pm SEM^a$		
Luteinizing hormone (ng MRC 69-104) ml	3.2-30.0	12.3 ± 1.3	16.0 ± 3.2	11.6 ± 1.2	13.7 ± 2.3	17.7 ± 1.5	n.s.
Total testosterone (ng/ml)	3.2-9.7	4.8 ± 0.3	5.9 ± 0.5	4.8 ± 0.2	5.6 ± 0.7	5.7 ± 0.3	n.s.
Free testosterone (pg/ml)	68-262	112 ± 9	135 ± 13	114 ± 8	128 ± 11	136 ± 8	n.s.

^{a}SEM = Standard error of the mean

patients who felt most anxious about sexuality (primary and secondary erectile impotence and premature ejaculation, group E_2) did not show decreased LH or androgen plasma concentrations.

As for frequency of sexual activity: although the patients described here reported decreased heterosexual activity, their total sexual activity, including masturbation, was not less than that of the normal controls. This is compatible with the fact that our patients did not complain of decreasing sexual desire. This latter fact may well explain the difference between our results and those of Legros and Raboch. Cooper et al (1970) described a group of patients suffering from 'constitutional impotence' which was characterized by low libido and decreased testosterone secretion in urine. Although Legros et al (1973) did not provide information on libido in their patients, Raboch et al (1975) reported that about half of their patients complained of decreasing sexual desire. Whether the decreased libido, which was probably accompanied by an impaired frequency of sexual activity (although data were not provided by the authors), was responsible for the decreased plasma testosterone levels, or whether a slightly impaired Leydig cell function may have contributed to the development of impotence, cannot be established. Our data so far indicate that psychogenic erectile impotence and premature ejaculation in men are not accompanied by changes in the pituitary testicular system, though the non-significant differences in gonadotrophic secretion may deserve further study.

Second Study

As already discussed, androgen hormones are necessary to maintain fully sexual activity in human males. It is generally accepted that hypogonadism brings about sexual dysfunction. There is, however, no detailed information available on the interaction of androgens and sexual behaviour in the range of subnormal plasma testosterone concentrations. In normal men these concentrations range from 3 to 10 ng/ml during the morning hours. Is the lower limit of the normal range identical with the threshold below which impairment of sexual function develops? Are there hypogonadal men with undisturbed sexuality? Answering these questions we may gain further insight into the role of androgens in sexual behaviour. We may also find a more adequate way of substituting androgens in hypogonadal patients. We report here on a study on 15 hypogonadal patients who were observed during periods with no medication, under placebo treatment, and with four different doses of testosterone (oenanthate).

Patients and design

Fifteen patients with hypogonadism gave their informed consent to participate in the study. The clinical data are given in Table 2. All patients had suffered from hypogonadism for more than two years and had been substituted previously with various doses of various androgen preparations. Androgen medication was stopped eight weeks prior to the beginning of

Table 2. Clinical data on 15 hypogonadal patients participating in the study on the role of testosterone in sexual behaviour

Patient	Age (years)	Permanent partner	Diagnosis	Plasma testosterone prior to substitution with testosterone (ng/ml)	Plasma LH (ng/ml)
(a) *Primary hypogonadism*					
1	53	yes	Loss of both testes at age 17	1.30	90.0
2	34	yes	XX-Male	1.26	46.5
3	37	yes	Subtotal loss of testes after trauma	2.02	110.0
4	38	yes	Klinefelter syndrome	2.16	43.0
5	31	yes	Testicular atrophy after orchitis	2.59	32.0
6	25	no	Klinefelter syndrome	3.00	61.0
7	30	yes	Klinefelter syndrome	3.13	45.0
8	38	yes	Testicular atrophy, cryptorchidism	3.51	29.0
9	37	yes	Testicular atrophy, cryptorchidism	3.53	42.0
(b) *Secondary hypogonadism*					
10	26	yes	Pituitary insufficiency of unclear origin	0.70	2.7
11	31	no	Hypothalamic hypogonadism	0.71	3.5
12	18	no	Pubertas tarda	0.69	3.1
13	27	no	Pubertas tarda	1.33	3.8
14	35	yes	Hypophysectomy because of pituitary tumour	1.57	4.8
15	53	yes	Hypothalamic hypogonadism	2.47	3.1

testosterone replacement within the study. There were six observation periods, each lasting one month. The first period (baseline) started four weeks after the previous androgen substitution had been stopped. In the second period the patients received an intramuscular injection of 25 mg Testoviron depot every two weeks. Testoviron depot consists of a mixture of testosterone propionate and testosterone oenanthate. In the third treatment period a placebo injection was given every two weeks. In the fourth period 50 mg, and in the fifth period 100 mg, were given twice a month. A sixth treatment period with twice 250 mg was employed only when the patients had not yet experienced sufficient improvement in their complaints. After the last intramuscular treatment period all patients received oral therapy with testosterone undecanoate (Andriol or Restandol, Organon). Doses ranged from 80 to 200 mg per day. The treatment schedule was revealed to the investigators who treated the patients but not to the patients themselves.

Each patient was given a diary. He was asked to fill in daily the number of spontaneous erections, frequency of masturbation, coitus and other sexual activities. For the evaluation of the data the total number of erections and ejaculations per treatment period has been calculated. The patients were seen every fortnight. At that time they filled in the Mood Scale (von Zerssen, 1976), two linear scales ranging from 'very bad' to 'very good' for 'I feel myself' and 'my partnership' and a linear scale ranging from 0 per cent to 100 per cent for 'my sexual drive'. For the evaluation of the data the distance in millimetres from the lower end of the linear scale to the mark of the patient has been calculated. For the sake of comparison the mean of the data of each of the four scales for each patient and treatment period has been used.

Blood was drawn during the morning hours at intervals of one week. Testosterone and LH were measured by radioimmunoassay as described above.

Results and discussion

The relation between sexual activity and plasma testosterone was analysed during the time when patients were without testosterone replacement. For this analysis we selected the phase of placebo treatment. Figure 1 shows the relation between the average plasma testosterone levels in each subject and the number of ejaculations which occurred during the placebo phase. The coefficient of correlation was $+0.405$ (not significant). The correlation between the average plasma testosterone and the frequency of erections was $+0.436$ ($P < 0.05$) during this phase. Since there was no significant difference between pretreatment phase and placebo phase with regard to sexual drive and the frequency of ejaculations and erections, it seems unlikely that the correlations mentioned are biased by placebo effects on sexual behaviour. Only two patients (11 and 13) reported no ejaculations at all. Both never underwent puberty (delayed puberty). It is remarkable that some patients with testosterone values below the lower limit of the normal range reported relatively high frequencies of ejaculation (Figure 1, patients 3 and 4).

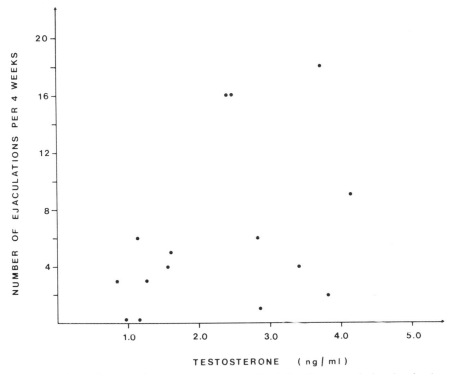

Figure 1. Relation between plasma testosterone and ejaculation frequency during the placebo phase.

Table 3 gives the average testosterone concentrations for all patients in each treatment period. For the periods during which testosterone was injected only those samples taken one week after the injections were considered, as these values fall approximately midway between the high values shortly after injections and the rather low values two weeks later and probably represent best the average testosterone concentrations available to the body. The patients rated their sexual drive on a linear scale. These data cannot be compared interindividually. The intraindividual comparison between different treatment phases (Wilcoxon test for paired data) showed no difference between the pretreatment period and the placebo phase. When the periods of testosterone treatment were compared with the placebo phase, a significant increase of the sexual drive was found only for the 100 and 250 mg phase ($P < 0.01$).

The influence of testosterone treatment on the frequency of ejaculations and of erections during the different phases is illustrated in Figure 2. We have considered the patients who reported a relatively high frequency of ejaculations during the pretreatment period — more than eight in four weeks — separately from those reporting eight or less ejaculations per four weeks. Neither group reported significantly different frequencies of

Table 3. *Average plasma testosterone concentrations in hypogonadal patients with and without testosterone substitution*[a]

	Mean (ng/ml)	Standard deviation	Probability
Pretreatment	2.15	0.25	n.s.
Placebo	2.10	0.30	
25 mg	3.05	0.21	<0.01
50 mg	3.95	0.22	<0.01
100 mg	5.70	0.33	<0.01
250 mg	9.05	0.74	<0.01

[a]Plasma levels were measured one week after intramuscular injection of testosterone oenanthate. Comparisons are made between placebo phase and each treatment phase.

ejaculation or erection in the pretreatment phase and in the placebo phase. The different treatment periods were again compared to the placebo phase by using the Wilcoxon test for paired observations. The patients who already had high ejaculation frequencies did not show an increase in the number of erections and ejaculations during the testosterone treatment periods. Those patients with low ejaculation frequencies, however, reported increases in the number of erections and ejaculations when treated with either 50, 100 or 250 mg testosterone; 25 mg had no effect. In the group with low ejaculation frequencies two subjects (12 and 13) with delayed puberty showed no increase of ejaculation frequency under testosterone treatment, although one of them reported the occurrence of erections under the highest testosterone dose.

The data obtained from the Mood Scale (von Zerssen, 1976) and from the linear self-rating scales 'I feel myself' and 'my partnership' were evaluated by comparing the placebo phase with the four periods of testosterone treatment using the Wilcoxon test for paired data. We tested all patients together, as well as the two groups with high and low frequency of ejaculations separately. No significant differences were found between the placebo phase and any of the testosterone treatment phases.

Our clinical experience and that of Davidson, Camargo and Smith (1979) suggest that the behavioural effects of testosterone injection in hypogonadal men, when they occur, are fairly rapid (i.e., in days rather than weeks); it is therefore likely that any therapeutic effect will be observed within a treatment period of four weeks. Since the evaluation of the testosterone effect on sexual behaviour relies mainly on the diaries filled out by the patients and not on interviews, the results ought not to be biased by the expectations of the investigator who treated the patients. When we look at the sexual behaviour of the hypogonadal patients during the pretreatment and the placebo periods, it appears that all patients — with the exception of two younger men with delayed puberty — reported ejaculations and erections despite very low testosterone values in some cases. The fact that so many of the hypogonadal patients had ejaculations in the period without substitution may be surprising. However, it has to be remembered that these data are based on subjective reports. Patients may record an orgasm as an ejaculation, even though only minute quantities of seminal fluid are ejaculated.

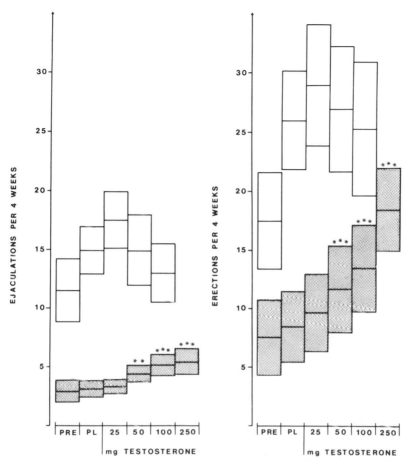

Figure 2. Erection and ejaculation frequencies in hypogonadal patients during the different phases of treatment. Mean values and standard errors of the mean are indicated. The white columns represent those patients who reported an ejaculation frequency greater than two per week during the placebo phase (n = 4). The stippled columns represent the patients who reported fewer than two ejaculations per week (n = 11). ** $P < 0.02$, *** $P < 0.01$ in comparison with the placebo phase.

Our data indicate that there is a wide individual variability in the threshold of plasma testosterone below which sexual function is impaired. This threshold varies from 2.0 to 4.5 ng/ml. Below the limit of 2.0 ng/ml all patients responded to testosterone substitution. Our observations further indicate that not every patient having testosterone values below the lower limit of the normal range (3.0 ng/ml) (Pirke and Doerr, 1975) needs substitution with testosterone. On the other hand there are patients with testosterone levels still in the normal range who do need substitution.

In the two patients with delayed puberty great amounts of testosterone were needed to increase the frequency of erections. It is not known what causes this effect. Changes in the metabolic clearance rate of testosterone do not seem to be responsible for this phenomenon, since the plasma levels of testosterone were as high as in other patients after substitution. The possibility exists that the sensitivity of target tissues to testosterone may be decreased. This assumption, however, is highly speculative.

CONCLUSION

The role of gonadal hormones in sexual behaviour of women remains uncertain. Endocrinological evaluation is therefore of little help in understanding the mechanisms of sexual dysfunction in the female. With the male the situation is different. Gonadal function should be evaluated for all patients with sexual dysfunctions in order to recognize patients with hypogonadism. In patients with psychogenic sexual dysfunctions the pituitary-gonadal function seems unaltered. It is therefore not surprising that these patients do not respond to androgen treatment (Benkert et al, 1979). In hypogonadal men an impairment of sexual disturbance develops when androgen supply drops below a threshold. This threshold may vary from patient to patient. An androgen substitution will improve sexual ability in hypogonadal men only when their testosterone levels are below their individual threshold.

REFERENCES

Anderson, D. C. (1974) Sex-hormone binding globulin. *Clinical Endocrinology,* **3,** 1-28.
Ansari, J. M. (1975) A study of 65 impotent males. *British Journal of Psychiatry,* **127,** 337-341.
Benkert, O., Witt, W., Adam, W. & Leitz, A. (1979) Effects of testosterone undeconoate on sexual potency and the hypothalamic-pituitary-gonadal axis of impotent males. *Archives of Sexual Behavior,* **8,** 471-479.
Bremer, J. (1959) *Asexualisation: A Follow-up Study of 244 Cases.* New York: Macmillan.
Carney, A., Bancroft, J. H. J. & Matthews, A. (1978) Combination of hormonal and psychological treatment for female sexual unresponsiveness. *British Journal of Psychiatry,* **132,** 339-346.
Comhaire, F. & Vermeulen, A. (1975) Plasma testosterone in patients with varicocele and sexual inadequacy. *Journal of Clinical Endocrinology,* **40,** 824-829.
Cooper, A. J., Ismail, A., Smith, C. G. & Loraine, J. A. (1970) Androgen function in 'psychogenic' and 'constitutional' types of impotence. *British Medical Journal,* **iii,** 17-19.
Cornu, F. (1973) *Katamnesen bei Kastrierten Sittlichkeitsdelinquenten aus forensisch-psychiatrischer Sicht.* Basel: S. Karger.
Davidson, J. M., Camargo, C. A. & Smith, E. R. (1979) Effects of androgen on sexual behavior in hypogonadal men. *Journal of Clinical Endocrinology and Metabolism,* **48**(6) 955-958.
Dittmar, F., Kockott, G. & Nusselt, L. (1977) Ein einfaches Instrument zur Messung von Gefuhlen, angewendet als Kriterium des Therapieerfolges bei Erektionsstorungen. In *Sexuelle Storungen* (Ed.) Kockott, G. pp. 116-122. Munchen: Urban & Schwarzenberg.
Fox, C. A., Ismail, A., Love, D. N., Kirkham, K. E. & Loraine, J. A. (1972) Studies on the relationship between plasma testosterone levels and human sexual activity. *Journal of Endocrinology,* **52,** 51-56.
Ismail, A., Davidson, D. W., Loraine, J. A. et al (1970) Assessment of gonadal function in impotent men. In *Reproductive Endocrinology* (Ed.) Irvine, W. J. pp. 138-147. Edinburgh: Livingstone.
Kraemer, H. C., Becker, H. B., Brodie, H. K. H. et al (1976) Orgasmic frequency and plasma testosterone levels in normal human males. *Archives of Sexual Behavior,* **5,** 125-132.

Kruez, L. E., Rose, R. & Jennings, R. (1972) Suppression of plasma testosterone levels and psychological stress. *Archives of General Psychiatry*, **26**, 479-482.

Langeluddecke, A. (1963) *Die Entmannung von Sittlichkeitsverbrechern.* pp. 82-85. Berlin: Walter de Gruyter.

Laschet, U. & Laschet, L. (1971) Psychopharmacotherapy of sex offenders with cyproterone acetate. *Pharmacopsyciatie*, **4**, 99-104.

Lawrence, D. M. & Swyer, G. J. M. (1979) Plasma testosterone and testosterone binding affinities in men with impotence, oligospermia, azoospermia, and hypogonadism. *British Medical Journal*, **i**, 349-351.

Legros, J. J., Franchimont, P., Palemvliers, M. & Servais, J. (1973) FSH, LH and testosterone blood level in patients with psychogenic impotence. *Endocrinologia Experimentalis*, **7**, 59-63.

Masters, W. H. & Johnson, V. E. (1970) *Human Sexual Inadequacy.* London: G. and A. Churchill.

Odell, W. D., Rayford, P. L. & Ross, G. T. (1967) Simplified, partially automated method for radioimmunoassay of human thyroid-stimulating growth, luteinizing, and follicle stimulating hormones. *Journal of Laboratory and Clinical Medicine*, **70**, 973-978.

Pirke, K. M. (1973) A comparison of three methods of measuring testosterone in plasma: competitive protein binding, radioimmunoassay without and radioimmunoassay including thin layer chromatoglraphy. *Acta Endocrinologica*, **74**, 168-176.

Pirke, K. M. & Doerr, P. (1975) Age related changes in free plasma testosterone, dihydrotestosterone and oestradiol. *Acta Endocrinologica*, **80**, 171-178.

Pirke, K. M., Kockott, G. & Dittmar, F. (1974) Psychosexual stimulation and plasma testosterone in man. *Archives of Sexual Behavior*, **3**, 577-584.

Raboch, J., Mellan, J. & Starka, L. (1975) Plasma testosterone in male patients with sexual dysfunction. *Archives of Sexual Behavior*, **4**, 541-545.

Santen, R. J. & Bardin, C. W. (1973) Episodic luteinizing hormone secretion in man: pulse analysis, clinical interpretation, physiologic mechanisms. *Journal of Clinical Investigations*, **52**, 2617-2628.

Skakkebaek, N. E., Bancroft, J., Davidson, D. W. & Warner, P. M. (1981) Androgen replacement with oral testosterone undecanoate in hypogonadal men; a double-blind controlled study. *Clinical Endocrinology*, **14**, 49-61.

Smith, K. D., Tcholakian, R. K., Chowdhury, M. & Steinberger, E. (1974) Rapid oscillations in plasma levels of testosterone, luteinizing hormone, and follicle-stimulating hormone in man. *Fertility and Sterility*, **25**, 965-975.

Schwartz, M. F., Kolodny, R. C. & Masters, W. H. (1980) Plasma testosterone levels of sexually functional and dysfunctional men. *Archives of Sexual Behaviour*, **9**, 355-366.

von Zerssen, D. (1976) with the cooperation of Koller, B. M. *Klinische Selbstbeurteilungs-Skalen* (KSb-S) aus dem Munchener psychiatrischen Informations-System (PSYCHIS-Munchen). Manual: Die Befindlichkeits-Skala. Weinheim: Beltz.

3

Hormones and the Sexuality of Women — the Menstrual Cycle

DIANA SANDERS
JOHN BANCROFT

INTRODUCTION

The role of hormones in determining the sexuality of women is of more than theoretical interest. Millions of women are receiving natural or synthetic steroids for one reason or another, and yet we know remarkably little about their behavioural effects. Hormone replacement in postmenopausal women is dealt with in Chapter 4. Here, we consider the woman during her fertile years. What is the connection between her menstrual cycle and her sexuality, and what are the likely effects of steroidal contraceptives on her behaviour?

The menstrual cycle is of interest, not only because it provides a recurring and predictable variation in sex steroids, but also because in most if not all other mammals there is a clear link between the female hormonal cycle and sexual behaviour. Is there any evidence of such a link in women, or has the human female evolved to such an extent that hormonal factors have become of negligible importance, overshadowed by other, psychological or social, mechanisms.

The animal model is a good starting point. Let us therefore look first at evidence from other species.

SEXUAL BEHAVIOUR AND THE HORMONAL CYCLE IN MAMMALS

It has long been recognized that for most species there are recurrent but short periods when the female is sexually receptive and usually more attractive to the male. This episodic sexiness is sometimes called 'heat'. Heape in 1900 was mainly responsible for introducing the term oestrus to describe this phenomenon. The term literally means 'in a frenzied state' and had previously been used to describe the gadfly (oestridae) which at certain stages in its life cycle drives cattle or horses into a state of frenzy. Eventually a clear link was established between this periodic sexual behaviour and the cyclicity of ovarian hormones. Such cycles were therefore called oestrous cycles and the principal ovarian hormones involved were termed oestrogens.

In mammals which menstruate (i.e., the Old World primates), the hormonal cycle is usually called the menstrual cycle, and as menstruation is the most obvious external indicator, the first day of menstrual bleeding is regarded as day 1 of the cycle. The majority of mammals do not menstruate, however, and for them the term oestrous cycle is used, with the oestrous behaviour being the most overt sign and the day when it first appears being called day 1 of the cycle. As we shall see, there are many varieties of cyclical sexuality which, whilst they have certain characteristics in common, also differ in many ways across species. What are the biological functions of cyclical sexual behaviour, and what mechanisms, hormonal or otherwise, control it?

The cycles of subprimate mammals vary considerably. Many mammals, such as sheep, goats or deer, are seasonal breeders. They are said to be seasonally polyoestrous, with long periods of 'anoestrus' during the spring and summer. Others have regular oestrous cycles until pregnancy occurs, though the length of the cycle varies. In virtually all subprimates studied, however, the function of the behavioural cycle is clear. Sexual activity is confined to a brief proportion of the animal's existence, closely linked to ovulation. In other words it is reduced to the minimum required to ensure reproduction and, in the case of seasonal breeders, its occurrence in the optimum season. In many species the biological advantages of this system are obvious; the sexually excited state is usually highly disadvantageous from most points of view; the animal is distracted and easy prey for predators or vulnerable to other dangers.

The hormonal mechanisms underlying such cyclical patterns are also very varied. Oestradiol is usually involved, but the temporal relationship between the oestradiol peak and oestrous behaviour varies from one species to another, as do the influences of other hormones. Progesterone is often important, but, for example, in the sheep the high level of oestrogen that provokes oestrous behaviour must have been preceded by a falling level of progesterone. In the rat the oestradiol peak must be followed by a sharp rise in progesterone if oestrous behaviour is to occur. In other species progesterone is not necessary at all. The precise mechanisms mediating between hormonal change and sexual behaviour are not fully understood but, for example, in the rat, the threshold for adopting lordosis in response to male mounting is lower during the oestrous phase. It is clear from hormone implantation experiments in the rat, cat and other non-primate species that direct effects of steroid hormones on central nervous system reactivity are involved. Also in the rat the extent of the genital sensory field varies according to the endocrine state, though it is not clear whether this is a central or peripheral effect or a combination of both (Komisaruk, 1978).

The attractiveness of the female to the male is also altered by hormone-induced mechanisms. The most obvious involve olfactory and visual cues. Olfaction is probably important in the sexual signalling system of most mammals, including primates, involving either urinary or vaginal odour (Keverne, 1978). The effects of such cues may involve specific and direct activation of the limbic system leading to sexual arousal or, less directly, the provision of information which with learning indicates that the female is receptive and hence worth approaching. (The 'releaser' effect of olfactory cues, the true pheromonal effect, when a complex behaviour pattern is triggered, is probably confined to insects.) In terrestrial primates visual cues are also important. Genital swelling at certain stages of the cycle may be obvious (e.g., chimpanzee) and clearly visible to the male from a distance. That this is not simply to provide a visual cue is suggested by the fact that obvious sexual swellings are more or less confined to those primates that live in multi-male troops (Clutton-Brock and Harvey, 1976). The direct effects of such genital changes on the female's behaviour may also be important. Heape (1900) wondered whether the 'congestion, stimulation or irritation of the copulatory organs . . . is in itself sufficient to induce oestrus or whether . . . other influences are essential'. Zuckerman (1932) considered it 'reasonable to surmise that when the sexual skin is swollen with oedema, its sensory nerve endings are stimulated by pressure and that this reflexly rouses the animal to sexual behaviour'. Such effects have received little attention from modern primatologists, but deserve further study. As such genital swellings are hormone dependent, this is further reason to believe that the behavioural effects of hormones may be mediated by peripheral (i.e., genital swelling) as well as central processes. We will return to this possibility when comparing primates with humans.

The varied nature of the determinants of cyclical sexual behaviour should now be clear. Not only does one have to consider peripheral as well as central mechanisms, but also the relative importance of the female and male in determining the pattern. This has usually been investigated by identifying three components of female sexuality: 'receptivity', the preparedness of the female to accept sexual mounting by the male, 'proceptivity', the extent to which the female will initiate and invite sexual contact, and 'attractiveness', non-behavioural characteristics of the female which increase the likelihood of the male's sexual approach. Each component may involve different hormonal mechanisms. Herbert (1977) and his coworkers have shown that proceptivity in oestrogen-treated oophorectomized Rhesus monkeys is androgen dependent, although Michael et al (1978) were unable to show any causal relationship between the rise in androgens and the increased proceptivity that both occur at mid-cycle. Oestrogens, whilst undoubtedly important for attractiveness and probably necessary for receptivity, may also play a role in proceptivity. Progesterone may have peripheral oestrogen-blocking effects on attractiveness as well as central effects of an inhibitory kind (Baum et al, 1977).

When considering primates we also find marked differences between species in the obviousness of the cyclical pattern. Whilst in some sexual activity is clearly confined to the periovulatory period, and is very similar in behavioural terms to the oestrous of many subprimate species, others show patterns which are by no means restricted to the fertile period although they are often maximal at that time. In certain circumstances such species may show sexual activity at any stage of the cycle. The cyclical pattern may be obscured by social and environmental factors, leading Yerkes (1939) to postulate that the extent to which the sexual activity of a species is linked to the female's hormonal cycle is inversely related to the degree of encephalization and the degree of sexual dominance of the female by the male. More recent evidence has shown Yerkes' hypothesis to be too simple. Whilst the dominance of the male is relevant, the degree of encephalization is less important than the level of sexual drive or the social structure typical of the species. In some instances it has been clearly essential for reproduction to link sexual activity with ovulation. In others, the level of sexual drive and hence the coital frequency is sufficient to ensure optimal fertility, so that the pattern of sexual activity can evolve to serve other biological purposes without jeopardizing reproduction. These points are well illustrated by comparison of three of the great apes: the gorilla, the orang-utan and the chimpanzee (Nadler, 1980; Short, 1981).

The male gorilla lives with a small harem of females. The huge size of the male is used to compete with other males to ensure access to such a group of females. But apart from his physical dominance, the male gorilla is a comparatively sexless creature with a very small penis and small testes relative to his body size. Sexual activity depends largely on the female taking the initiative. This she does around the time of ovulation, though for most of her fertile life she will be in a state of lactational anoestrus. Even with a group of females, there will be relatively long periods between occasions when one of the group is sexually receptive, proceptive, and presumably attractive. Between these times, the male appears to be sexually uninterested. It is obviously essential in such circumstances that sexual activity occurs around the time of these occasional ovulations if the group is to reproduce.

The orang-utan has a very different social structure. These apes live predominantly in isolation, presumably because of the constraints of their food supply. Adult males inhabit a 'home range' which may overlap with that of one or more females. The male orang-utan is not only much bigger than the female but also, by comparison with the gorilla, more highly sexed. If he comes across a female he is likely to copulate with her, 'raping' her if she is not receptive. The females, who usually live with one or two dependent young, tend to keep clear of the males. As with the gorilla, their periods of fertility are widely spaced, presumably because of lactational anoestrus, but when they are once again fertile they will seek out a male and make themselves sexually available. The male reveals his position by his characteristic vocalizations.

Nadler's studies of the captive orang-utan have been informative for a variety of reasons. In his earlier studies (Nadler, 1977) he reported that pairing male and female orang-utan in a typical experimental setting led to copulation more or less every time and regardless of the phase of the female's menstrual cycle. He did find, however, that around the time of ovulation, copulation was more likely to be repeated and the female would be more receptive and less needing to be 'raped'. In later experiments (Nadler, 1980) he gave the female control over access to the male by putting her in an adjoining cage with a connecting opening large enough for her to pass through but too small for the male. He then found that the female would visit the male and copulate with him around the time of ovulation.

This is a parallel to the situation in the wild. This evidence illustrates very clearly how a natural pattern can be obscured by studying behaviour in an unnatural setting. Thus we see that the female orang-utan shows a clear oestrous cycle, linked to ovulation, providing that she is able to control access to the male.

The chimpanzee is quite different again, living in small social groups of both males and females. Whereas sexual activity may occur at any time in the female's cycle, it is undoubtedly maximal for a period of 8 to 16 days when there is considerable swelling of the female's external genitalia, clearly visible to males from some distance. During this phase there is frequent mating with most males in the group. This genital swelling is associated with the rising oestradiol levels of the follicular phase and ovulation occurs towards the end of this period of maximal swelling or early in the following phase of detumescence. Most of the copulation during this phase is therefore unlikely to lead to conception. It is nevertheless possible that this pattern is serving the sexual needs of the males in the group without weakening group cohesion. It may also help the female to select a mate for reproductive purposes. There is a tendency, towards the end of the phase of maximal swelling for the female to disappear from the rest of the group in the company of one particular male. According to Tutin (1980) conception is most likely to result from these temporary consortships. Here then we have an oestrous pattern of a different kind, much more extensive than is required for reproduction alone but possibly serving other needs of a social group of highly-sexed animals.

Thus we can conclude that the various combinations of male physical dominance and high sexual drive will result in less clear oestrous patterns if the male has access to the female. Social organization, on the other hand, may either give the female more control of sexual activity, in which case the periovulatory pattern will be more obvious, or lead to other patterns of sexual activity which are serving social in addition to reproductive purposes.

A further factor to be considered is novelty. If the male and female are not used to one another, sexual interest in each other is likely to be enhanced, obscuring the influences of the hormonal cycle. In many experiments involving laboratory animals this factor has not sufficiently been taken into consideration. A cyclical pattern may become more apparent once the effects of novelty have declined. This is particularly relevant to the expression of proceptivity in the female. If she is sufficiently attractive to the male, perhaps because of novelty, there will be no need to show proceptive behaviour. Once her attractiveness wanes, her proceptivity may increase to compensate and then reveal a cyclical proceptive pattern. This is especially relevant to those primates, such as the marmoset or humans, who normally cohabit in stable pairs.

Before turning to the human female, we therefore need to note that in some primates non-hormonal factors may override or obscure the hormonally determined cyclical pattern. Furthermore in certain cases, perhaps because optimum fertility has been maintained, sexual behaviour has evolved to serve other non-reproductive functions. We should expect such factors to be even more important in the human.

THE MENSTRUAL CYCLE AND SEXUALITY IN WOMEN

Available evidence on the distribution of sexuality during the human menstrual cycle is somewhat conflicting, though in general there is little to support a mid-cycle or periovulatory peak. In a recent review of 32 studies, 17 found increased sexual activity premenstrually, 18 postmenstrually, four during menstruation and only 8 around the time of ovulation (Schreiner-Engel, 1980). There are a number of reasons to account for these discrepant findings. The method of identifying the periovulatory phase is likely to be crucial for recognizing a mid-cycle pattern. Identifying a temporal relationship with menstruation is much easier and less likely to be inaccurate. Udry and Morris (1977) have shown that by varying the method of timing ovulation, one can produce a variety of behavioural patterns using the same data. Also, the incidence of anovulatory or otherwise endocrinologically abnormal cycles is sufficiently high to be a problem if not identified (Doring, 1969; Metcalfe, 1979; Metcalfe and MacKenzie, 1980). It is therefore important to determine ovulation and other characteristics of the cycle by means of hormonal measurement.

A second important issue relates to the methods of recording sexual behaviour. Many studies have relied on retrospective accounts which not only are notoriously unreliable, but may also tend to emphasize recall of behaviour linked to clear events such as menstruation, spuriously indicating a perimenstrual pattern. There has also been a tendency to use vague definitions of behaviour or sexuality such as 'libido' or 'sexual gratification' and a failure to distinguish between behaviour which is initiated by the female (i.e., proceptive) or by the male. One recent study did make a useful attempt to identify female-initiated behaviour, including masturbation and the use of erotic fantasy or literature, and reported a peak of such behaviour around ovulation (Adams, Gold and Burt, 1978). However, this study can be criticized on other grounds; the methods used to identify the time of ovulation were unreliable and a reinterpretation of the data failed to show this mid-cycle peak (Kolodny and Bauman, 1979).

So far, very few studies have combined hormonal and behavioural assessment through the cycle. Persky, O'Brien and Kahn (1976) and Abplanalp et al (1979) divided the hormonal cycle into three and five phases, respectively, using hormonal markers. In neither study were any differences in behavioural parameters found between cycle phases, though the numbers involved were small (11 and 14 women respectively). In a larger study, involving 55 women with normal ovulatory cycles, careful assessment of mood and sexuality was carried out using daily diaries (Sanders, 1981; Sanders et al, 1983; Bäckström et al, 1983; Bancroft et al, 1983). Based on frequent blood-sampling (two or three times weekly), each cycle was divided into six hormonally distinct phases called early, mid and late follicular and early, mid and late luteal (see Figure 1). Menstruation occurred in the early follicular and ovulation during the late follicular phase. The women were divided into three groups. One-third had presented at a gynaecological clinic complaining of premenstrual syndrome (PMS). One-third were volunteers who reported PMS but had not sought medical help for it. One-

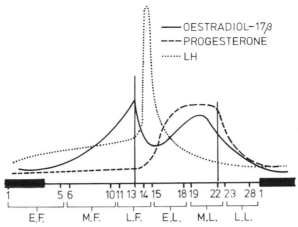

Figure 1. Cycle phase division: six hormonally distinct phases of the menstrual cycle shown for a standard 28-day cycle. E.F., M.F., L.F. − early, mid and late follicular: E.L., M.L., L.L. = early, mid and late luteal (Sanders, 1981).

third were relatively free from premenstrual symptoms. Thus it was possible to study women with and without cyclical mood change. Most of the subjective ratings of mood and sexuality were highly correlated with one another and were therefore subjected to a principal components analysis. This allowed 76 per cent of the variance to be expressed in four summary variables or components. The first component accounted for 43 per cent of the variance and all of the variables loaded on it positively or negatively. This was labelled 'well-being' and showed a marked cyclical pattern in the clinic group and the volunteers with PMS but not in the remainder (Figure 2). It was found that approximately a third of the variance of the subjective sexual ratings was involved in this component, indicating that those women who experienced an improvement in well-being in the follicular phase and a deterioration during the luteal phase showed a comparable pattern in their sexual feelings. This is not surprising — sexuality is much more likely to be expressed when one is feeling generally well and energetic — but it is a fact that has not been taken into consideration in previous studies. Premenstrual symptoms are common (Andersch, 1980). The discrepancies in results mentioned previously may reflect different proportions of women with marked premenstrual syndrome in different studies.

In our study, sexual activity involving the partner showed a cyclical pattern with a significant peak in the mid follicular phase (i.e., post-menstrual, not periovulatory). Some of the women in the study indicated whether they or their partners initiated sexual activity. Initiation by the woman or mutually by both partners was also more likely to occur in the mid follicular phase. There was a non-significant tendency for initiation by the partner to be more frequent during the luteal phase (Bancroft et al, 1983). The fourth component in the principal components analysis reflected sexual feelings independent of general well-being and contrasted with

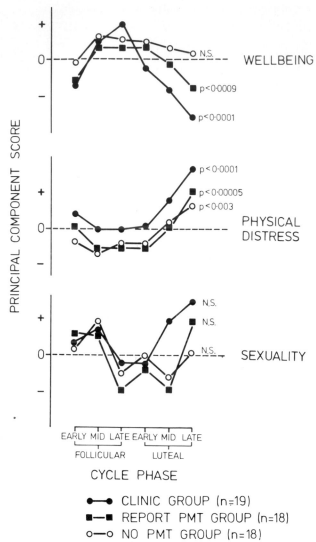

Figure 2. The principal components of subjective variables showing cyclical changes in three groups of women. For the 'sexuality' component the pattern was significant ($P < 0.01$) for the three groups combined but not separately (Sanders et al, 1983). (PMT (premenstrual tension) = PMS.)

self-rated energy. This component was called 'sexuality' and also showed a peak in the mid follicular phase and a further peak during the late luteal phase (see Figure 2) (Sanders, 1981).

Thus in this study, except for a general tendency for sexuality to vary with general well-being, we found no evidence of a mid-cycle or periovulatory peak. There was, however, definite evidence of a mid follicular (i.e., post-menstrual) increase in interest and activity and, to a lesser extent, a late luteal (premenstrual) increase in sexual interest.

Consistent evidence of a different kind has recently been reported by Schreiner-Engel et al (1981a). Using photometry they measured the vaginal blood flow response of 33 women to erotic stimuli in the laboratory at three different stages of the menstrual cycle, early to mid follicular, periovulatory and mid to late luteal. Although the cycle phases were established by counting back and forwards from menstruation, they were confirmed by hormone assay. Blood flow responses during the follicular and luteal phases were significantly higher than those in mid-cycle (see Figure 3).

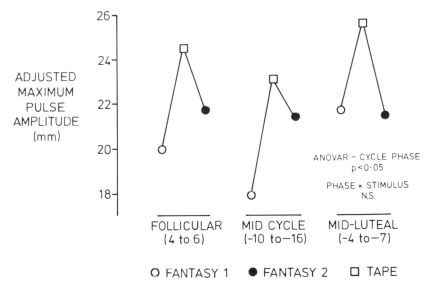

Figure 3. Vaginal response to erotic stimuli at three phases of the menstrual cycle in 33 normal women. Three stimuli (two fantasy and one audio tape) were used on each occasion. There was a significant difference in degree of response between the three cycle phases, with the mid-cycle response being lowest (Schreiner-Engel et al, 1981a).

The weight of evidence, both of subjective and objective indices of female sexuality, is therefore in favour of a perimenstrual rather than a periovulatory pattern, though it should be emphasized that this pattern is a subtle one, easily obscured by other factors. What are the possible explanations for this seemingly paradoxical finding? Are there non-biological factors that could account for it, and should we assume that it is fundamentally different from the patterns commonly found in the subhuman primates?

Menstrual abstinence

It has long been assumed that pre- and postmenstrual peaks of sexual activity are products of a period of abstinence during menstruation. Taboos on sexual activity during menstruation are widespread (Ford and Beach, 1957; Martin and Long, 1969). Even with the more 'enlightened' attitudes to bodily function that prevail in our society today, there are many women and possibly even more men who are reluctant to have intercourse during menstrual flow. (Sometimes, with heavy bleeding, this is inevitable, but in many cases the blood loss is sufficiently slight to be of no practical consequence.) Thus it is assumed that anticipation of menstrual abstinence accounts for the premenstrual increase and cessation of abstinence the postmenstrual increase in sexual activity. Gold and Adams (1978) have presented some data to support this view and obviously it accords with common sense. In our opinion, abstinence is likely to contribute to the perimenstrual pattern but is not a sufficient explanation. It is not unusual to find women whose sexual interest or preparedness to engage in sexual intercourse is restricted to a brief period of the cycle. They sometimes present this as a problem. This pattern is comparable to that observed in subhuman primates, such as the gorilla, where both male and female sexual interest is generally low. The difference is that whereas in the gorilla this coincides with ovulation, in such women the peak is nearly always peri-menstrual. It is difficult to account for that pattern on the basis of abstinence in view of the long periods of unenforced abstinence for the rest of the cycle.

In the study of Schreiner-Engel et al (1981a) described above, vaginal response to erotic stimuli in the laboratory was greater in the mid follicular and mid luteal phase than at mid-cycle. It could be that after a period of sexual abstinence a woman will show more response to erotic stimuli, but not in anticipation of abstinence.

Avoidance of conception

The time around menstruation is relatively infertile and this fact might increase the likelihood of sexual activity. However, one would expect this to affect sexual intercourse rather than sexual interest, whereas in our study both showed a similar pattern. Also, no difference was found between those women using 'safe' methods of contraception (i.e., sterilization or IUCD) who would be less affected, and those using less safe (i.e., barrier) methods, which being more intrusive, might also focus more attention on the possi-bility of conception. It is therefore unlikely that concern about fertility could account for this observed cyclical pattern.

The non-specific effects of well-being

We have already emphasized the effects of cyclical mood change on female sexuality. In those women where it is marked, there will be a tendency to maximize sexuality in the mid and late follicular phases. But this would not account for the sexual peak being confined to the mid follicular phase as most measures of well-being are maximal in the late follicular phase, and it would certainly not account for any premenstrual increase in sexuality. It may, however, account for some of the mid-cycle peaks reported in the literature.

Perceptual and other psychological changes

Studies of taste, touch, smell, hearing and response to visual stimuli indicate that general perceptual sensitivity is increased in the follicular phase (Henkin, 1974). This again will contribute to a late follicular rather than mid follicular peak of sexuality. Breast sensitivity, however, does increase markedly during the luteal phase and through menstruation (Robinson and Short, 1977; see Figure 4). In many women this is associated with unpleasant breast tenderness and is an important component of the premenstrual syndrome, but in some women these changes could enhance erotic awareness and contribute to a premenstrual peak of sexuality. There is no evidence of genital swelling around ovulation as found in some primates, but pelvic congestion does occur during the perimenstrual period and this may lead to enhanced genital and sexual awareness. This could well contribute to the perimenstrual peak of sexuality, though the hormonal or physiological mechanisms are likely to be different to those determining the mid-cycle swelling of primates.

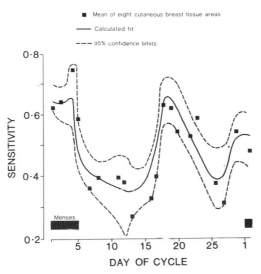

Figure 4. Changes in tactile sensitivity of the breast in a nulliparous woman during a normal menstrual cycle. (Reproduced from Robinson and Short, 1977, with kind permission of the authors.)

The role of hormones

It is difficult to see how changing oestradiol levels could account for this perimenstrual pattern, and there has been a consistent failure to find correlations between oestradiol and female sexuality (Persky et al, 1978b; Bancroft et al, 1983; Schreiner—Engel, personal communication 1981). The importance of oestradiol for women is emphasized in Chapter 4 by Dennerstein & Burrows, but the amount required for normal female sexuality is likely to be low and fluctuations of oestradiol above that level are probably irrelevant. This is comparable to the role of testosterone in men (see Chapter 2).

The role of progesterone is even more obscure. It is possible that it has an inhibitory effect which reduces female sexual interest or responsiveness during the luteal phase. If so, the premenstrual decline in progesterone might account for the perimenstrual increase in sexuality. No evidence to support this was found by Bancroft et al (1983) although Schreiner-Engel (personal communication 1981) did find her measures of sexual responsiveness to show increasingly negative correlations with progesterone as the cycle proceeded. More evidence is therefore needed before these uncertainties can be resolved. It has also been suggested that the luteal phase progesterone decreases the attractiveness of the female to the male (Udry, Morris and Waller, 1973), but in our study (Bancroft et al, 1983) male-initiated behaviour was marginally greater in the luteal than in the follicular phase, as if to compensate for a decrease in female interest.

The general role of testosterone in female sexuality is considered in more detail later in this chapter, but could the cyclical change in androgens account for the perimenstrual pattern of female sexuality? There is a predictable rise in testosterone and androstenedione during the normal menstrual cycle, reaching their highest levels during the late follicular and early luteal phases (see Figures 5, 6) (Vermeulen and Verdonck, 1976; Bäckström et al, 1983). This pattern is a mirror image of the pattern of sexuality already described (see Figure 7). Obviously no immediate effect of testosterone on sexuality is occurring, except possibly a negative one, but could this pattern be due to a delayed effect of testosterone? In hypo-gonadal men the sexual effects of testosterone replacement take several days or a week to become noticeable, and reach a maximum usually in about two weeks (Skakkebaek et al, 1981). If a similar time relationship operated in women, then the mid-cycle rise in testosterone could produce behavioural effects around menstruation. In the study of Schreiner-Engel et al (1981a) the cyclical changes in vaginal responsiveness were related to testosterone levels. The overall pattern observed by them (see Figure 3) was more

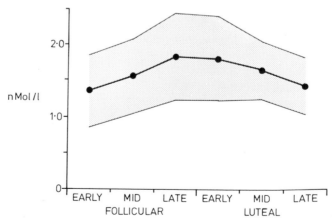

Figure 5. Plasma testosterone levels (mean ± 1 SD) for six phases of the cycle in 36 women with normal menstrual cycles (Bäckström et al, 1983).

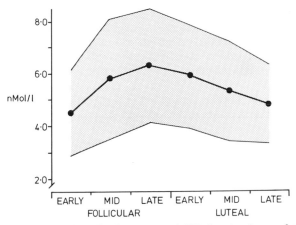

Figure 6. Plasma androstenedione levels (mean ± 1 SD) for six phases of the cycle in 34 women with normal menstrual cycles (Bäckström et al, 1983).

marked in women with relatively high testosterone levels, and, in particular, the response in the mid luteal phase was positively correlated to plasma testosterone. Further evidence is required, but it remains a possibility that testosterone contributes to the perimenstrual pattern of human female sexuality.

At the present time, it is therefore necessary to keep an open mind about the determinants of this pattern. But what function could it serve? The human primate is a highly-sexed species. The female, living usually in a stable relationship with the male, normally experiences more than enough sexual activity to ensure optimum fertility. It should be remembered that optimum fertility is not necessarily the same as maximum fertility. Short

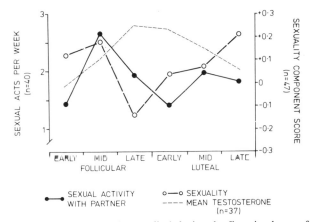

Figure 7. Levels of sexual activity and 'sexuality' during the first six phases of the cycle contrasted with the mean levels of testosterone. 'Sexuality' is the principal component score (see Figure 2). Details of testosterone levels are shown in Figure 5 (Bancroft et al, 1983).

(1982) has recently summarized the contrast between so called r and K selection. The r-selected species reproduce maximally at all times, whereas the K-selected species has a rate of reproduction which is related to the carrying capacity of the habitat. Too many offspring is maladaptive, and such species, including humans and the great apes, require adequate birth spacing for optimum survival. This is achieved in part by lactational anoestrus, but in the human it may also have been facilitated by separating maximum sexual activity from ovulation. There may be other evolutionary advantages of such a pattern. Cyclical female sexuality could have a re-inforcing effect on the male-female pair bond, countering the otherwise dulling effect of habituation. However, if such an advantage is to operate the pattern should not at the same time increase the likelihood of further pregnancies with their inevitable interruption of the sexual relationship.

Should the human female be regarded as fundamentally different in this respect from other animals? It may be that the human species is the only one that can afford to separate the time of maximum sexuality from ovulation. But apart from this there is sufficient variation amongst other species in these patterns and their underlying mechanisms to allow the human female to take her place amongst the rest of the animal kingdom. Obviously the sexuality of women is affected by many factors which are uniquely human, but we do not have to deny our biological heritage completely.

The Effects of Oral Contraceptives

One incontrovertible effect of oral contraceptives is that the normal hormonal cycle is radically altered. Ovulation is usually inhibited, follicular development may occur to a variable extent, but the luteal rise in progesterone is unlikely. At the same time there is a cyclical pattern of exogenous steroids with both synthetic oestrogen and progestagen being maintained at a relatively stable level for 21 days and then falling sharply and remaining negligible for the next seven days until the next pill cycle starts. If the normal hormonal cycle has any relevance to the usual pattern of femal sexuality, then we might expect a different pattern with women on the pill.

Before considering such cyclical consequences, is there any evidence that steroidal contraceptives have a more general effect on female sexuality? Unfortunately the literature on this important subject is confused and it is difficult to draw any firm conclusions. Several large scale studies (e.g., Westoff, Bumpas and Ryder, 1969) have shown that the frequency of coitus was higher in women on the pill than in those using other methods of contraception or no method at all. Whilst this does indicate that widespread negative effects of oral contraceptives on female sexuality are unlikely, there are difficulties in interpreting such evidence. First, women who choose oral contraceptives may be different sexually from those who prefer other methods. Secondly, in a cross-sectional study one is mainly observing women who find oral contraceptives acceptable. It is difficult to know how many women start on the pill and give it up because of sexual side-effects. Thirdly, coital rates tell us little about the quality of sexual experience.

Adoption of an effective method of contraception may remove obstacles to the male's sexual demands; coital frequency might therefore increase even with a reduction in the woman's spontaneous interest or enjoyment.

According to a large general practice survey (RCGP 1974), women using oral contraceptives are approximately four times more likely to complain of sexual difficulties than women using other methods. Once again, caution is required in interpreting such evidence. The provision of oral contraception provides a better opportunity for talking about sexual problems than most other reasons for attending the general practitioner.

The problem is further complicated by the relationship between mood and sexuality, already mentioned earlier in relation to the normal cycle. Grant and Pryse-Davies (1968), in their early study of the effects of oral contraception, made combined ratings of depression and loss of libido and found the combination to be adversely affected the higher the progestagen content. Kutner and Brown (1972) found the opposite; pills containing high doses of progestagen were associated with less severe depression. Once again, a selection factor might be operating, with women susceptible to depressive reactions being less likely to stay on such pills. Herzberg et al (1971) found that women who stopped the pill because of loss of libido were more depressed than those who continued. Cullberg (1972), in one of the better studies, compared three oestrogen/progestagen combinations with a placebo. He found the active pills produced more psychological side-effects than the placebo, but the incidence and severity of these side-effects did not vary with the progestagen dose. Sexual impairment was slight in this study and he concluded that when it occurred it was secondary to mood change. Cullberg also made the interesting observation that the adverse emotional reactions were most likely in those women with a previous history of pre-menstrual syndrome. Relevant evidence is lacking, but it may well be that the majority of women with PMS are unable to tolerate oral contraceptives and are less likely to be found amongst pill-using populations (e.g., Andersch, 1980).

The direct effects of the constituents of oral contraceptives on female sexuality therefore remain uncertain and await further evidence. One possibility that has been explored is that the circulating androgens are lowered by oral contraceptives, with resulting adverse sexual effects. To investigate this possibility, 20 women complaining of sexual problems that were attributed to oral contraceptives were compared with 20 women on the same pills but free from sexual problems. There was no difference between the two groups in their androgen levels, though in both groups testosterone and androstenedione were low and SHBG relatively high (see Figure 8). Further negative evidence from this study was the failure to obtain sexual improvement in the problem group by giving additional androstenedione.

What happens to the cyclical pattern of female sexuality in women using oral contraceptives? Udry, Morris and Waller (1973) compared women taking oral contraceptives with those taking a placebo. Whilst there was no difference in overall sexual activity in the two groups, there was some evidence of a different pattern through the cycle. Women on placebo tended to show a decline in sexual activity during the luteal phase which was not

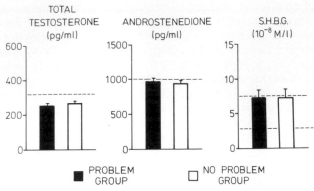

Figure 8. Mean plasma testosterone, androstenedione and SHBG levels in two groups of oral contraceptive users: 20 women with sexual problems (problem group) and 20 women without sexual problems (no problem group). (Four weekly samples from each subject.) (Bancroft et al, 1980.)

apparent in the pill-taking group. Adams, Gold and Burt (1978) found a peak of female-initiated sexual activity in the first four or five days of the pill cycle, whereas with non-pill-using women there was a noticeable peak nearer the mid-cycle.

In our experience, women on oral contraceptives often report feeling most sexually interested towards the end of the pill-free week (Bancroft et al, 1980). In relation to menstrual bleeding, this is comparable to the post-menstrual peak of the normal cycle but is clearly different from the endocrine point of view. At this stage the endogenous steroids in many women are beginning to escape from the control of the previous pill cycle and there is a rise in oestradiol-17β and testosterone which usually reaches a peak during these first few days of the next cycle before control is regained. In some women this behavioural pattern is sufficiently marked to present a problem, with sexual interest and enjoyment being confined to this brief phase of the pill cycle. Figure 9 shows such a pattern in a particular woman with the behavioural change closely related to the peaks of endogenous oestradiol and testosterone. It is tempting in such cases to attribute the lack of sexuality at other times in the cycle to the pill-induced suppression of oestradiol-17β or testosterone, but so far, in a small number of such women, we have been unable to alter this pattern by increasing either the oestradiol-17β or the testosterone, whereas in each case stopping the pill or lowering the progestagen content has produced beneficial results. Further evidence is needed on this important point. A study comparing women on triphasic and combined preparations, currently in progress, should throw light on the possible role of the pill constituents.

The Role of Androgens in Women

For many years testosterone has been regarded as the 'libido hormone' in women, as in men, though the evidence has been largely anecdotal or based on highly unphysiological evidence (e.g., Waxenburg, Drellich and

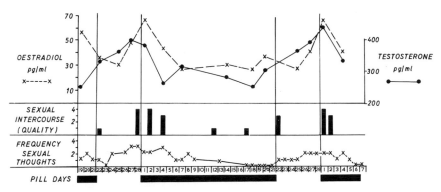

Figure 9. Cyclical changes in sexuality and endogenous sex steroids in one woman on oral contraceptives (Ovranette).

Sutherland, 1959). This view has been reinforced by the finding that pro-captivity in female rhesus monkeys is, at least in part, androgen dependent (Herbert, 1977), though as mentioned earlier this has been disputed.

Carney, Bancroft and Mathews (1978) reported the first controlled evidence of the effects of androgens on the sexuality of women. Sexually unresponsive women showed more improvement after sexual counselling when it was combined with testosterone than when combined with diazepam. This was taken as evidence of a sexually enhancing effect of testosterone in women. However, two further studies (Mathews, Whitehead and Kellet, 1983; Dow, 1982 personal communication) failed to support this conclusion. Using a similar design involving counselling but comparing testosterone with placebo rather than diazepam, they found no difference between testosterone and placebo. This makes it likely that the observed differences in the first study were due to a negative effect of diazepam on the counselling rather than to a positive effect of testosterone. Nevertheless, there has been some evidence linking testosterone and female sexuality. In a group of 11 women Persky et al (1978a) found a positive association between mid-cycle testosterone level and frequency of sexual activity throughout the cycle. In the study of oral contraceptive users (Bancroft et al, 1980), a significant positive correlation was found between mean plasma testosterone and ratings of sexual interest, but only in those women free from sexual problems. This reminds us of the important possibility that hormone-behaviour relationships may be obscured by psychological factors.

When we return to the two recent studies of the menstrual cycle (Schreiner-Engel et al, 1981a, b; Bancroft et al, 1983) a more complex but intriguing picture starts to emerge. We have already considered the possible delayed effect of testosterone on cyclical female sexuality. It is also possible that such androgenic effects operate on a time scale that precludes them from appearing predictably in a 28-day cycle. It would then be more appropriate to look for tonic rather than cyclical effects, and to do this we examined the association between average or mid-cycle testosterone levels and average levels of sexuality throughout the cycle. Such correlations are shown in Table 1. An important distinction is between women who masturbate and those who don't. In the former, there was a high correlation between testosterone and frequency of masturbation, but no correlation with frequency of sexual activity with the partner or with sexual feelings. For the women who didn't masturbate, the latter correlations tended to be negative, significantly so where sexual feelings were concerned. Presumably factors other than testosterone determine which women masturbate, as the two groups had similar testosterone levels (means of 453 ng/ml for the masturbators and 476 ng/ml for the non-masturbators). Psychological and social factors are likely to be important in this respect.

Table 1. *Correlations between mid-cycle testosterone and various aspects of sexuality (from Bancroft et al, 1982)*

	Sexual feelings	Frequency of sexual activity with partner	Frequency of masturbation
Women who masturbate (n = 21)	−0.05	−0.1	0.79[++]
Women who do not masturbate (n = 15)	−0.44[+]	−0.26	—

[+] $= P < 0.05$
[++] $= P < 0.01$

In the study of Schreiner-Engel et al (1981a, b) a comparable picture emerged. Vaginal response to erotic stimuli in the laboratory was positively correlated with testosterone levels, but when women with high and low testosterone were compared, the high group reported more problems and dissatisfaction with their sexual relationship and less frequent sexual activity or sexual desire.

In both studies, therefore, sexuality which was independent of a relationship (i.e., masturbation or response to erotic stimuli) was positively associated with testosterone, but sexual aspects of relationships had negative associations. How can we account for this seeming paradox?

In our study (Bancroft et al, 1983) there was also an association between testosterone level and lifestyle. Women who were married or cohabiting had lower testosterone levels than those living alone. Women working full-time had higher testosterone than those who were working part-time or as 'housewives'. These differences were small (reaching only 10 per cent level of significance), but they were consistent with those of Purifoy and Koopman (1980) who found an association between testosterone levels and professional roles in American women. The possibility that such testosterone levels are a consequence rather than a cause of the lifestyle has to be considered. However, the consistent evidence linking exposure to androgens during early female development with career orientation and a relative rejection of conventional female roles (Ehrhardt and Meyer-Bahlburg, 1979) indicates that androgens can have an influence, and this could well be the case in our subjects. This being so, one can postulate that testosterone is associated with personality development and adoption of lifestyles which are in conflict with conventional female heterosexuality, thus accounting for the paradoxical findings in these two studies.

If, in spite of the sexually enhancing effects of testosterone, other effects produce heterosexual dissatisfaction or conflict, one might predict that a proportion of women so affected would adopt homosexual lifestyles. In that way their testosterone-induced sexuality would not be in conflict with their testosterone influenced personalities. It is therefore of some interest that in several studies of lesbian women about one-third have had relatively high testosterone levels (see Chapter 5 by Meyer-Bahlburg). If this hypothesis is correct, then it is difficult to see how 'normal' female sexuality is dependent on androgens. However, we should not assume that testosterone-induced female sexuality is unphysiological or unnatural. It may simply conflict with the prevailing social norms of femininity, representing a powerful biological reason for modifying those norms. As yet, this hypothesis is based on limited data, but it has implications of profound importance, and there is certainly a need for further evidence of this kind. In the meantime, it is worth pointing out that biological evidence does not necessarily favour the social status quo.

REFERENCES

Abplanalp, J. M., Rose, R. M., Donnelly, A. F. & Livingston-Vaughn, L. (1979) Psycho-endocrinology of the menstrual cycle. II. Relationship between enjoyment of activities, moods and reproductive hormones. *Psychosomatic Medicine,* **41,** 605-615.

Adams, D. B., Gold, A. B. & Burt, A. D. (1978) Rise in female sexual activity at ovulation blocked by oral contraceptives. *New England Journal of Medicine,* **299,** 1145-1150.

Andersch, B. (1980) Epidemiological, hormonal and water balance studies on premenstrual tension. *Thesis. University Göteborg.*

Bäckström, T., Sanders, D., Leask, R., Davidson, D., Warner, P. & Bancroft, J. (1983) The relationship between mood change and hormone levels during the menstrual cycle in women with premenstrual syndrome and normal volunteers. *Psychosomatic Medicine* (in press).

Bancroft, J., Davidson, D., Warner, P. & Tyrer, G. (1980) Androgens and sexual behaviour in women using oral contraceptives. *Clinical Endocrinology,* **12,** 327-340.

Bancroft, J., Sanders, D., Davidson, D. & Warner, P. (1983) Sexuality during the menstrual cycle and the role of androgens. *Psychosomatic Medicine* (in press).

Baum, M. J., Everitt, B. J., Herbert, J. & Keverne, E. B. (1977) Hormonal basis of proceptivity and receptivity in female primates. *Archives of Sexual Behavior,* **6,** 173-192.

Carney, A., Bancroft, J. & Mathews, A. (1978) Combination of hormonal and psychological treatment for female sexual unresponsiveness: a comparative study. *British Journal of Psychiatry,* **133,** 339-346.

Clutton-Brock, T. H. & Harvey, P. H. (1976) Evolutionary rules and primate societies. In *Growing Points in Ethology* (Ed.) Dateson, P. P. G. & Hinde, R. A. pp. 195-237. Cambridge: University Press.

Cullberg, J. (1972) Mood changes and menstrual symptoms with different gestagen/estrogen combinations. *Acta Psychiatrica Scandinavica* (Supplement 236)

Doring, G. K. (1969) The incidence of anovular cycles in women. *Journal of Reproduction and Fertility* (Supplement 6), pp 77-81.

Ehrhardt, A. A. & Meyer-Bahlburg, H. F. L. (1979) Psychosexual development: an examination of the role of prenatal hormones. In *Sex, Hormones and Behaviour. Ciba Foundation Symposium* 62 (New Series). Amsterdam: Excerpta Medica.

Ford, C. S. & Beach, F. R. (1957) *Patterns of Sexual Behaviour.* New York: Harper & Row.

Gold, A. R. & Adams, P. B. (1978) Measuring the cycles of female sexuality. *Contemporary Obstetrics & Gynecology,* **12,** 147.

Grant, E. C. G. & Pryse-Davies, J. (1968) Effect of oral contraception on depressive mood changes and on endometrial monoamine oxidase and phosphatases. *British Medical Journal,* **iii,** 777-780.

Heape, W. (1900) The 'sexual season' of mammals and the relation of the 'pro-oestrus' to menstruation. *Quarterly Journal of Microscopical Science,* **44** (New Series), 1-70.

Henkin, R. I. (1974) Sensory changes during the menstrual cycle. In *Biorhythms and Human Reproduction* (Ed.) Ferin, M., Hallberg, F., Richart, R. M. & Vande Wiele, R. L. New York: Wiley.

Herbert, J. (1977) The neuroendocrine basis of sexual behaviour in primates. In *Handbook of Sexology* (Ed.) Money, J. & Musaph, H. Amsterdam: Excerpta Medica.

Herzberg, B. N., Draper, K. C., Johnson, A. L. & Nicol, G. C. (1971) Oral contraceptives, depression and libido. *British Medical Journal,* **iii,** 495-500.

Keverne, E. B. (1978) Olfactory cues in mammalian sexual behaviour. In *Biological Determinants of Sexual Behaviour* (Ed.) Hutchison, J. Chichester: Wiley.

Kolodny, R. C. & Bauman, J. E. (1979) Letter to Editor. Female sexual activity at ovulation. *New England Journal of Medicine,* **300,** 626.

Komisaruk, B. R. (1978) The nature of the neural substrate of female sexual behaviour in mammals and its hormonal sensitivity: review and speculations. In *Biological Determinants of Sexual Behaviour* (Ed.) Hutchison, J. Chichester: Wiley.

Kutner, S. J. & Brown, W. L. (1972) Types of oral contraceptives, depression and premenstrual symptoms. *Journal of Nervous and Mental Disorders,* **155,** 153-162.

Martin, C. B. & Long, E. M. (1969) Sex during the menstrual period. *Medical Aspects of Human Sexuality,* **3,** 37-49.

Mathews, A., Whitehead, A. & Kellett, J. (1983) Psychological and hormonal factors in the treatment of female sexual dysfunction. *Psychological Medicine* (in press).

Metcalfe, M. G. (1979) Incidence of anovulatory cycles in women approaching the menopause. *Journal of Biosocial Science,* **11,** 39-48.

Metcalfe, M. G. & Mackenzie, J. A. (1980) Incidence of ovulation in young women. *Journal of Biosocial Science,* **12,** 345-352.

Michael, R. P., Richter, M. C., Cairn, J. R., Zumpe, D. & Bonsall, R. W. (1978) Artificial menstrual cycles, behaviour and the role of androgens in female Rhesus monkeys. *Nature,* **275,** 439-440.

Nadler, R. D. (1977) Sexual behaviour of captive orang-utans. *Archives of Sexual Behavior,* **6,** 457-475.

Nadler, R. D. (1980) Determination of sexuality in Great Apes. In *Medical Sexology* (Ed.) Forleo, R. & Pasini, W. Amsterdam: Elsevier/North Holland.

Persky, H., O'Brien, C. P. & Kahn, M. A. (1976) Reproductive hormone levels, sexual activity and moods during the menstrual cycle. *Psychosomatic Medicine,* **38,** 62-63.

Persky, H., Lief, H. I., Strauss, D., Miller, W. R. & O'Brien, C. P. (1978a) Plasma testosterone level and sexual behavior of couples. *Archives of Sexual Behavior,* **7,** 157.

Persky, H., Charney, N., Lief, H. I., O'Brien, C. P., Miller, W. R. & Strauss, D. (1978b) The relationship of plasma estradiol level to sexual behavior in young women. *Psychosomatic Medicine,* **40,** 523-535.

Purifoy, F. E. & Koopmans, L. H. (1980) Androstenedione, T and free T concentrations in women of various occupations. *Social Biology,* **26,** 179-188.

Robinson, J. E. & Short, R. V. (1977) Changes in human breast sensitivity at puberty, during the menstrual cycle and at parturition. *British Medical Journal,* **i,** 1188-1191.

Royal College of General Practitioners (1974) *Oral Contraceptives and Health.* London: Pitman.

Sanders, D. (1981) Hormones and behaviour during the menstrual cycle. *Ph.D. Thesis, University of Edinburgh.*

Sanders, D., Warner, P., Bäckström, T. & Bancroft, J. (1983) Mood and the menstrual cycle. *Psychosomatic Medicine* (in press).

Schreiner-Engel, P. (1980) Female sexual arousability: its relation to gonadal hormones and the menstrual cycle. *Ph.D Thesis, New York University.*

Schreiner-Engel, P., Schiavi, R. C., Smith, H. & White, D. (1981a) Sexual arousability and the menstrual cycle. *Psychosomatic Medicine,* **43,** 199-214.

Schreiner-Engel, P., Schiavi, R. C., Smith, H. & White, D. (1981b) Plasma testosterone and female sexual behavior. *Proceedings of the 5th World Congress of Sexology* (Ed.) Hoch, Z. & Lief, H. I. Amsterdam: Excerpta Medica (in press).

Short, R. V. (1981) Sexual selection in man and the Great Apes. In *Reproductive Biology of the Great Apes* (Ed.) Graham, C. E. pp. 319-341. London: Academic Press.

Short, R. V. (1982) The biological basis for the contraceptive effects of breast feeding. In *Breast Feeding and Fertility Regulation.* WHO publication (in press).

Skakkebaek, N., Bancroft, J., Davidson, D. & Warner, P. (1981) Androgen replacement with oral testosterone undecanoate in hypogonadal men: a double blind controlled study. *Clinical Endocrinology,* **14,** 49-61.

Tutin, C. E. G. (1980) Reproductive behaviour of wild chimpanzees in the Gombe National Park, Tanzania. In *The Great Apes of Africa* (Ed.) Short, R. V. & Weir, B. J. *Journal of Reproduction and Fertility* (Supplement 28), pp 43-57.

Udry, J. R. & Morris, N. M. (1977) The distribution of events in the human menstrual cycle. *Journal of Reproduction and Fertility,* **51,** 419-425.

Udry, J. R., Morris, N. M. & Waller, L. (1973) Effect of contraceptive pills in sexual activity in the luteal phase of the human menstrual cycle. *Archives of Sexual Behavior,* **2,** 205-214.

Vermeulen, A. & Verdonck, L. (1976) Plasma androgen levels during the menstrual cycle. *American Journal of Obstetrics and Gynecology,* **125,** 491-494.

Waxenburg, S. E., Drellich, M. G. & Sutherland, A. M. (1959) The role of hormones in human behavior. I. Changes in female sexuality after adrenalectomy. *Journal of Clinical Endocrinology & Metabolism,* **19,** 193-202.

Westoff, C. F., Bumpas, L. & Ryder, N. B. (1969) Oral contraception, coital frequency and the time required to conceive. *Social Biology,* **16,** 1-10.

Yerkes, R. M. (1939) Sexual behavior in the chimpanzee. *Human Biology,* **ii,** 78-111.

Zuckerman, S. (1932) *The Social Life of Monkeys and Apes.* London: Kegan Paul, Trench & Trubner.

4

Hormone Replacement Therapy and Sexuality in Women

LORRAINE DENNERSTEIN
GRAHAM D. BURROWS

INTRODUCTION

Sexuality reflects a complex interaction of biological, sociocultural and psychological factors. The last two factors play an increasingly prominent role in the sexual behaviour of primates, especially in the human. Whilst much is known of the role of gonadal hormones in animal sexual behaviour, the effect of hormones on human female sexuality is the subject of much controversy. This is somewhat surprising when one considers that many million women are receiving steroidal contraceptives or postmenopausal hormone replacement therapy.

Any role of gonadal hormones in sexuality is of obvious clinical significance for women who have reached the stage of ovarian hormonal deficiency. Whilst the life expectancy of women has increased over the last four generations, there has been no matching prolongation of gonadal endocrine activity. The menopausal decline in ovarian function now occurs earlier relative to the total life span.

An increasing number of women experience a surgical menopause somewhat earlier than the mean age of the natural menopause of 50 years. In the USA in 1975 725 000 hysterectomies and 471 000 oophorectomies were performed, more than half on women under 45 years of age (Zussman et al, 1981).

With changing expectations of sexuality women now hope to enjoy sexual relationships well into their later years. For both women and their physicians the two clinically important questions are: (1) Are any changes in sexual behaviour to be expected with hormone depletion at the menopause? (2) What effects do hormone replacement therapies have on sexual response? This chapter will review the available evidence and discuss the clinical implications which follow.

ANIMAL STUDIES

Endocrine influences on sexuality are more prominent in lower mammals where sexual behaviour has been shown to vary predictably with the phases

Clinics in Endocrinology and Metabolism — Vol. 11, No. 3, November 1982.
0300-595X/82/11.03/661 $03.00 © 1982 W. B. Saunders Company Ltd

of the reproductive cycle. Consideration of these hormonal effects provides some interesting hypotheses as to the possible modulatory roles of hormones in the human.

Non-Primates

The sexual behaviour of non-primates has been investigated in field and laboratory studies. Sexual receptivity in the non-primate female mammal is usually measured by observation of the mammal assuming lordotic posture (Davidson, 1972). Field studies provide much information about mating patterns and the possible influence of social factors. Laboratory studies have enabled changes in sexual behaviour to be correlated with actual hormonal events. Environmental factors can be kept constant and hormonal events manipulated. The effects of hormones on sexual behaviour were elucidated using techniques which involved extirpative surgery at specific times in the reproductive cycle. The behavioural response without a particular hormone was then evaluated and compared with behaviour consequent on replacement of the hormone (Davidson, 1972).

The regulation of sexual behaviour by hormones in female non-primates was reviewed by Feder (1977). Spontaneously ovulating female non-primates typically showed sequential activation of the various tissues involved in reproduction (genital, hypophyseal, neural). The steroid hormones most significant for maintaining cycles of sequential activity of these tissues were oestrogen and progesterone. Oestrogens (particularly oestradiol-17β) were found to activate female sexual behaviour in a wide variety of non-primate species. The effect of progesterone on sexual behaviour varied among species studied. In rodents, such as rats, hamsters and guinea pigs, oestrogen secretion preceded a rise in pre-ovulatory progesterone which had a facilitatory action on sexual behaviour. In ewes, a period of luteal progesterone secretion prepared tissues for the activating effect of oestrogen. It appeared that under normal conditions progesterone probably had little or no role in the activation of sexual behaviour in cows, dogs and rabbits. Exogenous progesterone was noted to have a biphasic action in some species (Dmowski, Luna and Scommegna, 1974). As well as the facilitatory action described above, progesterone was found to suppress female sexual behaviour in certain species (e.g., guinea pigs) if given before oestrogen had had an adequate period of time to prepare the tissues.

Primates

Many species of female primates show discrete menstrual cycles and mate throughout the cycle. Both Old and New World monkeys show changes in behaviour during the female reproductive cycle. The role of hormones in the sexual behaviour of primates was reviewed by Herbert (1977). Copulation was found to be most likely to occur near mid-cycle and least likely in the luteal phase. Michael and Bonsall (1977) used an operant conditioning technique in which females had to press a lever 250 times to gain access to males. Shortest mean access time coinciding with highest ejaculate frequency occurred during reverse cycle days 18 to 16, one day after the oestradiol peak. Longest times were at the beginning and end of the cycle. Individual and social factors were found to modify sexual behaviour more frequently than in non-primates. The sexual behaviour of primates was consequently somewhat less predictable than that of sub-primate species (Herbert, 1977).

Oophorectomy of monkeys was found to reduce sexual interaction with males, although to varying degrees and not in all species. Administration of oestradiol-17β stimulated sexual receptivity and increased the female's attractiveness to the male. Progesterone given to oestrogen-treated females resulted in a a decline in their sexual receptivity and attractiveness to males (Herbert, 1977). Dmowski, Luna and Scommegna (1974) reported that oophorectomized monkeys when administered androgens also displayed increased attempts to solicit mounting from males. Caution is needed in interpreting the possible role of androgens in female sexual behaviour as it is known that androgens are the precursors of oestrogens in the ovary, testis, brain and peripheral tissues. Peripheral conversion of androgens to oestrogens occurs at a rate of 1.0 to 1.5 per cent. This conversion rate is significant considering the difference in the biological activity per unit of mass of these steroids. Central neuroendocrine tissues aromatize androgens. Aromatization was most active in the preoptic area and hypothalamic nuclei, tissues long known to be of importance in sexual behaviour (Naftolin et al, 1975). Hence it has been suggested that androgens first undergo conversion to oestrogens and only in the latter form affect sexual behaviour. In support of this hypothesis is the claim that dihydrotestosterone, androsterone and chlortestosterone, compounds that do not undergo conversion to oestrogens, fail to induce sexual receptivity (Dmowski, Luna and Scommegna, 1974). A specific effect of androgens on female sexual behaviour is suggested by findings that removing adrenals from oophorectomized monkeys causes them to remain unreceptive and sexually unattractive to males even when administered oestradiol. Receptivity is restored by testosterone or androstenedione (Herbert, 1977). Some workers have attributed the mid-cycle peak of proceptivity and receptivity to testosterone, which also rises at this time. Michael and Bonsall (1977) showed that a normal pattern of sexual behaviour could be produced in oophorectomized monkeys by replacing oestradiol and progesterone in doses that produced near physiological levels. The addition of testosterone in physiological doses made no difference to sexual behaviour. They noted that when testosterone had stimulated female sexuality in earlier studies, it had been administered in dosages 15 to 400 times that needed for physiological levels and had produced plasma androgen levels similar to those of males. Androgen-induced sexual behaviour may be blockaded by pretreatment with anti-androgens. Antiandrogens such as cyproterone acetate have been found to block central and peripheral androgen actions. These substances are without oestrogen effects and may inhibit aromatization of androgen to oestrogen (Naftolin et al, 1975).

Mechanism of Action

Neuroendocrine. The central neural sites of action of hormones in mammals have been determined by techniques of intracerebral implantation of hormones in oophorectomized animals or by surgical lesions to cerebral areas. The administration of radioactively-labelled hormones has enabled the localization of sites at which hormones are concentrated within the central nervous system. These experiments have demonstrated that hormones affect sexual behaviour when applied to certain hypothalamic areas (Everitt, 1977).

The way in which hormones affect the central nervous system has not been ascertained. One hypothesis is that hormones may alter neural activity by directly or indirectly modulating monamine neurotransmitter activity. This subject was recently reviewed by Everitt (1977). Pharmacological studies suggest that serotonin (5-hydroxy-tryptamine), dopamine and adrenaline have inhibitory effects on sexual behaviour in female rats, while it has been suggested that noradrenaline is excitatory. During the oestrus cycle, after castration and following treatment with sex hormones, alterations in the levels of serotonin, dopamine and noradrenaline were observed in various areas of the brain. These alterations could reflect effects on synthesis, uptake or breakdown. Kamberi and Kobayashi (1970) have demonstrated that monoamine oxidase activity changes cyclically in the hypothalamus and amygdala of the female rat. Anatomical investigations show similarity of sites in the brain where (1) implants of hormones induce sexual activity, (2) steroid uptake can be demonstrated, and (3) monamine cell bodies and terminals are present in abundance.

Pheromones. Another important mechanism of action of hormones relates to the way in which behaviour of another animal is affected by the secretion of hormone-dependent pheromones. Pheromones are chemical substances which are secreted in minute quantities by one organism and which act through the olfactory processes of another member of the same species to modify behaviour. Olfactory signalling persists over time, allowing information to be transmitted even in the absence of the signalling animal. There are three kinds of responses to pheromones among mammals (Keverne, 1977). Primer pheromones alter the physiology and consequent behavioural repertoire of the releaser animal. The response is slow to develop and requires prolonged stimulation. Olfactory imprinting may occur at a critical stage in neonatal development in some mammals. Releaser pheromones such as the sex attractants produce a more or less immediate change in the behaviour of the recipient.

Observation under field and laboratory conditions suggests that olfactory cues are important in the sexual behaviour of various species such as the rat, mouse, hamster, dog, cat and ungulates (Keverne, 1977). Michael, Keverne and Bonsall (1971) demonstrated the presence of a hormone-dependent vaginally-secreted pheromone in rhesus monkeys. The sex attractant, identified from vaginal secretions, was a series of short-chain aliphatic acids which, when applied to the sex skin area, elicited male sexual response to previously unattractive (oophorectomized) females. The effectiveness of these pheromones in stimulating male rhesus monkey sexual behaviour varied between individuals, with social conditions, and with the type of behaviour stimulated. Keverne (1977) reported that rendering males temporarily anosmic did not impair the males' response to familiar oestrogenized females but prevented their response to other oestrogenized females. These findings emphasize the effect of learning and that pheromonal activity in many species is not that of the stereotyped behaviour elicited in insects.

Pheromones are present in vaginal and underarm odours of humans. In some cultures body odours are regarded as erotic, particularly those arising from the woman's genitalia. In Western society there is often considerable effort to avoid or disguise body odours with deodorants and perfumes. The role of pheromones in sexual behaviour of the human is unclear.

Methodological Considerations

There are obvious methodological differences between studies of animal sexual behaviour and that of humans which limit comparison of findings. Whalen (1966) summarized the three major difficulties. Firstly, human sexuality is usually inferred from subjective reports, whereas animal sexual behaviour is deduced from direct observation and measurement of discrete components of behaviour. Laboratory studies of human sexual behaviour are only a recent phenomenon, being pioneered by Masters and Johnson (1966). They provide valuable physiological information but by their very nature impose restrictions on the type of study possible. Secondly, investigators of human behaviour tend to discuss sexuality using motivational terms such as 'libido' while animal behaviour researchers discuss sexuality in response terms, such as lordosis. This leads to comparison of non-analogous facets of human and animal sexuality. Thirdly, the motivational terms used to describe human behaviour are ambiguous. The term 'libido' is widely used but rarely defined. Freud defined libido as the energy of the sexual instinct. Libido referred specifically to the force of sexual desire rather than to pleasure or gratification from sex (Freud, 1905). Later workers have used the term more generally so as to embrace any aspect of sexual response from orgasm to absence of discomfort during intercourse (Cullberg, Gelli and Jonssen, 1969).

THE EFFECTS OF DEPLETION OF OVARIAN
HORMONES ON HUMAN SEXUALITY
Natural Menopause

Epidemiological studies seek to demonstrate whether a sudden change in sexuality occurs at the menopause, or whether there is a steady change with increasing age. Kinsey et al (1953) noted a decline with age in incidence and frequency of marital coitus, and of coitus to the point of orgasm. A decline was not evident for solitary activities of women, such as masturbation or nocturnal dreams to orgasm, until well after 60 years of age. In Kinsey's study, 48 per cent of the women who had experienced a natural menopause believed that their sexual response had decreased at this time. Somewhat surprisingly, such changes were attributed by Kinsey either to aging changes in the male or to the opportunity for women to use the excuse of menopause for discontinuing sexual relationships in which they were never particularly interested. Kinsey concluded that there was little evidence of any effect of aging on female sexuality until late in life.

Conflicting evidence is provided in later studies. Pfeiffer, Verwoerdt and Davis (1972) showed a dramatic decline in the sexual interest of women between the years of 45 and 55. A parallel decline in male sexual interest was not evident. Hällström (1977) also found dramatic declines in the sexual interest, capacity for orgasm and coital frequency of women in the middle years of life. A fundamental question is whether the observed decrease in sexuality was related to a progressive decline due to chronological aging or to the menopause. Hällström (1977) was able to demonstrate that decreased sexual function was significantly associated with menopausal status rather than age. While recognizing that considerable individual variations existed, Hällström noted that the majority of the postmenopausal women reported impairment of their sexual interest during the previous five years.

Aetiology of changes in sexuality at the menopause

Are behavioural changes at the menopause due to endogenous hormonal changes or to the psychological or social factors important during this life phase? The theories advanced to explain behavioural changes include:

Hormonal. Changes are attributed to declining ovarian function. The behavioural changes may reflect a change in brain, in particular hypo-thalamic function, with changing levels of steroids. The endocrine changes responsible for the symptoms may be lowered levels of oestrogens, progesterone, or both, or raised levels of follicle-stimulating hormone and luteinizing hormone. Alternatively symptoms could reflect an imbalance elsewhere in the hypothalamic-pituitary-gonadal axis.

Mood changes and sexual disinterest are sometimes claimed to be secondary manifestations of disabling vasomotor symptoms such as hot flushes and sweating (Lauritzen, 1973). The vasomotor symptoms and those of atrophic vaginitis are held by some to be the only 'true' symptoms of ovarian failure (Utian, 1972).

A hormonal basis is suggested by the epidemiological studies which have demonstrated changes in sexuality occurring directly in relation to this phase of declining hormone production. There is also evidence for a hormonal aetiology from the results of studies of hormone 'replacement' therapy. These studies are reviewed later.

Hormonal factors as causes of sexual decline were noted by Masters and Johnson (1966). Oestrogen deficiency may result in atrophic vaginal changes and consequent physical discomfort, pain at coitus and lessening of sexual interest. While women with decreased sexual interest were more likely to suffer from external dyspareunia, no direct relationship was evident between impairment of sexual interest and urinary total oestrogens (Hällström, 1977).

Psychological. Most psychological theories focus on loss. Deutsch (1945) referred to the loss of reproductive capacity as 'a partial death'. The depletion and decline in sexual attractiveness, usefulness and biological function was experienced by some women as loss with resulting depression.

Declining sexual interest may occur secondarily to depressed mood. Hällström (1977) found a significant association of declining sexual interest with the Hamilton Rating Score of Depression and also with the personality trait of introversion (Eysenck Personality Inventory).

The importance of premorbid personality has been emphasized. Benedek (1950) claimed a better outcome for women whose 'adaptive capacity has not been exhausted by previous neurotic processes'. Hällström (1977) found that women who had enjoyed sex in younger years were more likely to maintain sexual response through the menopause.

Sociological. Sociological menopausal changes may be culturally defined and engendered. Women in many cultures attain increased status and enjoy greater freedom with the menopause. In these cultures the achievement of the menopause is rewarded. Flint (1975) found that Indian women who experienced cultural gains on attaining menopause experienced fewer menopausal problems. In contrast, in Western cultures the menopause appears to be a sign of decline. This is emphasized by the usage of the term 'climacteric' which literally refers to something or somebody being around the top of the ladder and starting on the way down (Benedek, 1950). Stresses necessitating social readjustments that occur at this phase of life include: adolescent rebellion and children leaving home, the arrival of grandchildren, the loss of youth and attractiveness in a youth-oriented society, the forced re-evaluation of expectations, death of parents, and increasing physical ill-health for the woman and her partner.

Role theorists stress the importance of woman's social role performance. The loss of a role, for example 'mothering', may be crucial in women who have few role alternatives, unless this is balanced by important cultural gains after menopause. Any consequent loss of self-esteem may result in depression. Van Keep and Kellerhals (1974) found fewer symptoms when children were still at home. Crawford and Hooper (1975) found more menopausal symptoms present when a daughter had married than when a son had married. Most vulnerable are said to be housewives experiencing maternal role loss who had overprotective or overinvolved relationships with their children (Bart and Grossman, 1978). Some behavioural scientists suggest that the answer to these problems is for women to structure alternatives for themselves and other women. Some American women's groups are working towards this end. Changes in women's roles may have already had some effect. Two recent studies (Schneider and Brotherton, 1979; Krystal and Chiriboga, 1979) have failed to confirm the importance of loss of parental role or the 'empty nest' syndrome.

Van Keep and Kellerhals (1974) found that women in the higher social class had fewer menopausal complaints. Higher social class was also found to be an important association with maintained sexual response at the menopause, as were the presence of positive, intact marriage relationships, high educational level and being employed (Hällström, 1977).

Surgical Menopause

Following removal of both ovaries there is a rapid change in hormonal profile and menopausal symptoms are usually more severe than those associated with the natural menopause (Studd, Chakravarti and Oram, 1977). Bilateral oophorectomy is nearly always performed in association with hysterectomy and the effect of this procedure must also be evaluated. This makes it difficult to assess the effects of bilateral oophorectomy. The operation of hysterectomy has apparently been associated with psychosexual sequelae since reports of its inception. One of the earliest accounts of hysterectomy was provided by Professor Giacomo Berengario da Carpi (1480-1550). He reports witnessing an operation in which his father removed a prolapsed gangrenous uterus. The patient lived for many years and was able to resume sexual relations with her husband, although there was absence of coital gratification (Ricci, 1943). Ellison (1964) wrote: 'among women there is a remarkable consistency in the belief that the removal of the uterus and the ovaries marks the end of sexual life, at least emotionally'. In studies where patients were asked specifically whether their sexual relations had changed after hysterectomy, the incidence of diminished sexual functioning varied from 10 per cent (Huffman, 1950) to 46 per cent (Studd, Chakravarti and Oram, 1977). This wide range of results reflects many variables. These may include the time interval since surgery (Utian, 1975), the inclusion of cancer patients in some studies (Drellich and Bieber, 1958), and differences in the preoperative psychological preparation of the patient for surgery. In studies where patients were reported to be well-informed about the nature of their operation, the incidence of subsequent sexual dysfunction was lower. Dodds et al (1961) found an incidence of 15 per cent, and Patterson and Craig (1963) noted sexual deterioration in 18 per cent.

Another confusing factor in the literature was that many of the samples reported were mixed, in that only some patients had undergone oophorectomy. Munday and Cox (1967), in an Australian study, found no correlation between sexual outcome and the conservation or destruction of ovarian function. This finding was confirmed by Utian (1975). He concluded that 'the operation of hysterectomy per se, irrespective of whether the ovaries were removed or not, is associated with a significant reduction of libido'.

The assessment of changes in sexual behaviour is superficial and limited in most studies. On some questionnaires only one item was asked about sexual behaviour. In the studies reported above, no attempt was made to define the type of alteration noticed by the patient or to determine whether the alteration was due to physiological or psychological factors.

A study carried out by the authors (Dennerstein, Wood and Burrows, 1977) aimed to identify any factors associated with the sexual dysfunction attributed to this operation. It was envisaged that this information would enable the development of clear guidelines to be established for prophylaxis and treatment. Eighty-nine women who had undergone hysterectomy and bilateral oophorectomy for benign causes were interviewed. Information was obtained relating to social, medical, gynaecological and psychological history, and a detailed sexual assessment was made. Each woman was asked about any changes in her sexual relations which she would attribute to the operation. Specific information was sought about changes in desire for sex, enjoyment of sex, vaginal lubrication, ability to reach orgasm, and painful sexual intercourse. Difficulties in the partner's sexual performance were specifically asked about.

Sexual relations were found to have deteriorated in 33 women (37 per cent), while 30 women (34 per cent) stated that their sexual relations had improved since the operation. Twenty-six (29 per cent) detected no change. The sexual morbidity incidence found was higher than that of the 28 per cent obtained in the earlier Australian study (Munday and Cox, 1967), but was similar to the incidence of 38 per cent found in a controlled study of general practice patients (Richards, 1974). Rather than focussing on the frequency of such sequelae, subjects were studied to determine which factors were associated with a poor sexual outcome.

The following factors were of interest with regard to sexual dysfunction. When oestrogens were not prescribed or were taken only sporadically, significantly more dyspareunia was found than when oestrogens were taken continuously. The presence of remembered preoperative anxiety concerning possible deterioration of sexual performance was associated with an overall deterioration of sexual relations after the operation. There was a significant relationship between the presence of this type of preoperative anxiety and subsequent loss of desire for sexual intercourse and increased dyspareunia. These results support a multifactorial aetiology of the sexual dysfunction found.

Most studies have been retrospective in nature. In the absence of pre-operative measures it cannot necessarily be presumed that the operation of hysterectomy did have such adverse effects. There have been two recent prospective studies. Martin, Roberts and Clayton, (1980) studied 49 randomly selected women awaiting hysterectomy for benign gynaecological conditions. A year after surgery 44 of these women were reassessed. Of 34 women with sexual partners, 11 reported an increase in sexual intercourse postoperatively, 19 reported no change, and four (13 per cent) reported a decrease. A prospective UK investigation by Gath, Cooper and Day (1981) studied 156 women before hysterectomy and six and 19 months post-operatively. Ninety-four per cent of women were seen at both follow-up assessments. There was no control group. At each assessment women were asked to rate the frequency and enjoyment of sexual intercourse on a five point scale. Eighty per cent of women had recovered their preoperative level of sexual activity by the fourth postoperative month. Six months after operation the reported frequency of intercourse was increased in 56 per cent of patients, unchanged in 27 per cent and decreased in 17 per cent. Reported enjoyment of intercourse was increased in 39 per cent, unchanged in 41 per cent and reduced in 20 per cent of women. Eighteen months after operation the findings were unchanged. As the sexual relationships of many of these patients must presumably have been already impaired by gynaecological disorders prior to the hysterectomy it is disappointing that so many failed to improve or worsened after the hysterectomy.

In summary, it would appear that the operation of hysterectomy adversely affects the sexual behaviour of some women. Oophorectomy in premenopausal women without adequate hormone replacement therapy is likely to have additional effects. The aetiology of the effects of hysterectomy and bilateral oophorectomy is likely to be multifactorial.

Psychological factors such as the symbolic meaning of the uterus and/or ovaries to the woman, her previous adaptation, and her expectations of surgery are all important. Prospective studies have found an unusually high incidence of psychiatric morbidity (55 to 57 per cent) in women awaiting hysterectomy (Martin, Roberts and Clayton, 1980; Gath, Cooper and Day, 1981). Biological factors must also be considered. Masters and Johnson (1966) noted that the orgasmic contractions by muscles in the outer third of the vagina are accompanied by rhythmic contractions of the uterus. Zussman et al (1981) noted that 'for some women, the quality of orgasm is diminished when these structures are removed'. Removal of ovaries additionally removes the gonadal hormones oestrogen, progesterone and androgens. Asch and Greenblatt (1977) have established that both premenopausal and postmenopausal ovaries produce significant quantities of androgens, perhaps as high as 50 per cent.

Few attempts have been made to directly correlate hormone levels with behavioural changes. Chakravarti et al (1977) studied endocrine changes and symptomatology after oophorectomy in 100 premenopausal women. They concluded that 'the known changes in the concentration of circulating steroids cannot be related directly to the occurrence of symptoms in individual patients, neither to the level of gonadotrophins, until more information is available on the biologically active functions of the circulating hormones and on their interactions with other factors'.

The possible role played by hormonal depletion may be studied by examination of clinical trials of hormone replacement therapy.

THE EFFECT OF HORMONE REPLACEMENT THERAPIES

Until recently the term hormone replacement therapy (or HRT) has been almost synonymous with oestrogen therapy. Recent concern about the long-term effects of unopposed oestrogen on the uterine endometrium (Smith, Prentice and Thompson, 1975; Ziel and Finkle, 1975) has prompted the addition of a progestogen for the last seven to ten days of the cycle for women who have not had hysterectomy. Progestogens have also been prescribed alone to relieve vasomotor symptoms of women for whom oestrogens are contraindicated (Bullock, Massey and Gambrell, 1975). Studd (1977) suggests the use of oestrogen and testosterone implants to restore libido to oophorectomized women. If changes in behaviour are due to declining ovarian hormone production then hormone therapy should alleviate these complaints. To provide evidence for this hypothesis, studies of hormone replacement therapy were reviewed. The only investigations considered were those which utilized double-blind placebo-controlled methodology, essential procedures to eliminate biases of both the investigator(s) and the subjects.

There have been few double-blind studies of the effects of androgens on sexual response and we could find no double-blind studies of the effects of androgens on postmenopausal women.

Few double-blind studies of oestrogen replacement therapy have measured changes in sexual response. Campbell (1976), in a placebo-controlled double-blind cross-over study, noted a significant improvement of vaginal dryness and improved coital satisfaction with conjugated equine oestrogen administration. There was no change in masturbation, orgasm, or coital frequency as measured by analogue scales.

Beneficial effects of oestradiol valerate were reported by Fedor-Freybergh (1977) on the following aspects of sexuality: libido, sexual activity, satisfaction, experience of pleasure, sexual fantasies, orgasm capacity, and sexual relevancy. An ordinal self-rating scale was used to measure sexual behaviour in this double-blind comparison study.

In the studies reviewed, several methodological problems influence the interpretation of the results. These include the inadequate description and definition of the women investigated in terms of endocrine status, making comparisons of results almost impossible. There is also the problem of defining and measuring the behavioural changes of the menopause. In many of the studies reported terms have been used in the 'lay' sense rather than with their clinical meaning. The varying measures may have produced some disparity.

There are the additional problems of differing drugs being used in varying doses. It is not known how long the effect of hormones may persist, and this may have modified the results of studies of short duration cross-over design.

Only one paper (Bullock, Massey and Gambrell, 1975) studied progestogen alone and this study was mainly concerned with assessing hot flushes. Further research into the effects of progestogens is needed.

The alleviation of behavioural changes by hormones does not indicate whether these symptoms were occurring as secondary phenomena to distressing vasomotor symptoms, also relieved by hormone administration (Lauritzen, 1973). A study of menopausal women who had no vasomotor symptoms helped clarify the aetiological role of hormones for behavioural changes at the menopause (Campbell, 1976). Fewer beneficial effects of oestrogens on psychological parameters were found than when the women studied also suffered vasomotor symptoms. Significant improvement in memory and anxiety scores were nevertheless evident, but there was no change with regard to any parameter of sexual function except for that of vaginal dryness. It is not clear whether these 20 women were endocrinologically as postmenopausal as the other women in the study.

Clinical Trial

With the exception of the relief of atrophic vaginal changes by oestrogen, contradictory findings were reported of the effects of hormone replacement therapy on sexuality. The basic problem was the lack of knowledge of the individual behavioural effects of oestrogen or progestogen.

A model used extensively in animal research involved investigation of sexual behaviour after oophorectomy and subsequent replacement therapy with oestrogen and progesterone. It was decided to utilize this model in order to investigate the effects of these hormones on human females (Dennerstein et al, 1980).

Sample. Women selected for study had undergone a hysterectomy and bilateral salpingo-oophorectomy for benign disorders and were aged less than 65 years. There was no past or present medical history making the use of oestrogen or progestogen inadvisable. In order to minimize the effects of psychological factors only women with stable and satisfying heterosexual relationships were chosen for study. It was thought that significant inter-personal conflicts or sexual dysfunction may overwhelm the effects of hormones.

Method. After initial assessment the women were randomly allocated to one of four medication groups: ethinyl oestradiol 50 μg; levonorgestrel 250 μg; ethinyl oestradiol 50 μg and levonorgestrel 250 μg — 'Nordiol'; placebo. All drugs were supplied as identical tablets (Wyeth). In the double-blind cross-over design used, each woman was to receive each compound daily for three months. If intolerable symptoms arose during a medication phase the woman was to be changed to the next drug in the sequence. During the study women were interviewed initially and monthly. Details of somatic, vasomotor, psychological and sexual variables were sought at interviews and rated on ordinal scales by the interviewer. Psychological assessments performed included the Eysenck Personality Inventory Form B, Hamilton Rating for Depression and visual analogue scales measuring mood, anxiety and sexual response.

Results. The 36 women who received all four drugs concurred significantly ($P < 0.001$) in their preference of the drug received. The order of preference was ethinyl oestradiol, 'Nordiol', norgestrel alone, and lastly placebo (Dennerstein et al, 1978a).

Interview reports of sexual desire, sexual enjoyment, and amount of spontaneous vaginal lubrication with coitus were recorded on an ordinal scale. Drugs were ranked and Figures 1 to 3 were drawn as histograms from the rankings. Increasing sexual desire, enjoyment and vaginal lubrication are shown as increasing ranks. Wilcoxon's matched pairs signed-rank test was used to test for differences between drugs. After the first month no statistically significant findings ($P < 0.05$) were evident. After the second month there was a significant difference between the oestrogen-containing compounds and the non-oestrogen-containing compounds for both sexual desire and enjoyment. The difference between norgestrel and the oestrogen-containing drugs was highly significant ($P < 0.01$) for sexual enjoyment. There was also significantly more vaginal lubrication reported after two months of ethinyl oestradiol therapy than after two months of placebo. After the third month ethinyl oestradiol was associated with significantly

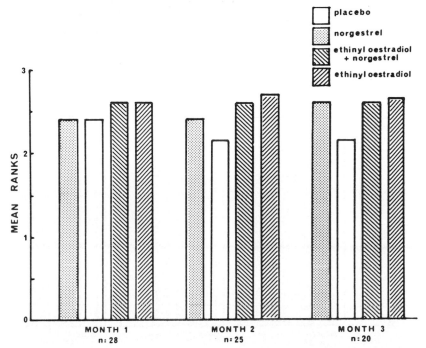

Figure 1. Hormone therapy and lubrication. From Dennerstein et al (1980), reprinted with kind permission from The American College of Obstetricians and Gynecologists. (*Obstetrics and Gynecology*, **56**, 316-322, 1980.)

more sexual enjoyment ($P < 0.05$) and desire ($P < 0.01$) than placebo. An interesting trend, although it is not statistically significant, was that during months one and two sexual enjoyment was lower with norgestrel alone than with placebo.

The frequency of orgasm was reported at monthly interviews. An analysis of variance was used to test for drug effects on orgasmic frequency. This method of analysis allowed a statistical determination of the separate effects of medication, patient differences, and the interaction between specific medication and individual patients to be evaluated. The results indicate that there was a significant difference between the various drugs on the frequency of orgasm. The highest number of orgasms occurred with ethinyl oestradiol, then 'Nordiol', then norgestrel, and the lowest number during placebo therapy. There was also a highly significant difference between individual patients in the frequency of orgasms experienced, and a highly significant patient-drug interaction, indicating that some women responded to different drugs in different ways.

An analysis of covariance was carried out to determine the proportion of the variance in orgasmic frequency that could be explained by the effect of hormones on hot flushes. The results demonstrate that the frequency of hot flushes also had a statistically significant effect on orgasmic frequency. As the magnitude of the effect of drugs on orgasmic frequency was

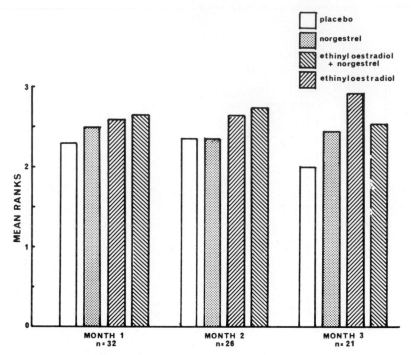

Figure 2. Hormone therapy and sexual desire. From Dennerstein et al (1980), reprinted with kind permission from The American College of Obstetricians and Gynecologists. (*Obstetrics and Gynecology,* **56,** 316-322, 1980.)

uninfluenced by including hot flush frequency as a covariate, the drugs appear not to affect orgasmic frequency by alleviation of hot flushes alone. A direct influence of the hormones on sexuality is suggested.

An analysis of variance was carried out on both daily and monthly reports of coital frequency. This showed no significant effects of the drugs administered on the frequency of intercourse. There were highly significant differences between patients and patient drug interactions with reported coital frequency. It was of interest that hormones significantly affected orgasmic frequency but not coital frequency. Coital rate is perhaps more likely to be influenced by the partner's wishes, whereas orgasmic frequency is more likely to reflect internal factors. These findings highlight the importance of distinguishing female from male sexual response.

The findings of a beneficial effect of oestrogen on sexual desire, enjoyment, vaginal lubrication and orgasmic frequency provide some evidence of effects of hormones in humans similar to those found in experiments with castrated primates.

CLINICAL IMPLICATIONS

The findings discussed above suggest that hormonal changes may affect sexual behaviour — at least in women with stable relationships. A

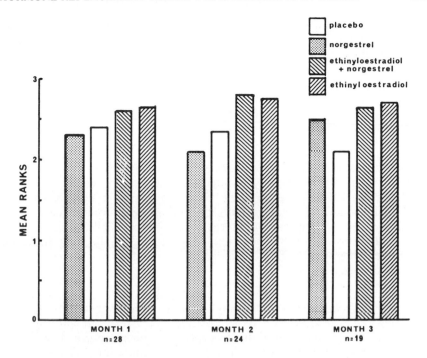

Figure 3. Hormone therapy and sexual enjoyment. From Dennerstein et al (1980), reprinted with kind permission from The American College of Obstetricians and Gynecologists. (*Obstetrics and Gynecology,* **56**, 316-322, 1980.)

deficiency of oestrogen may not necessarily be the cause of sexual problems presenting in mid-life, but may provide a biological vulnerability which for women with a somewhat tenuous sexual adjustment may be enough to tip the balance from 'just coping' to sexual dysfunction. Once sexual dysfunction exists it is unlikely that mere administration of oestrogen will produce a sufficient change in sexual behaviour to reverse the dysfunction because of the profound psychological effects, including those of learning and the development of performance anxieties. Other interventions may be needed.

All women presenting with sexual dysfunction after a natural or artificial menopause should receive a careful assessment which may involve history and examination of both the woman and her partner. Assessment is aimed at delineating the problem, the level of psychosexual development of the woman and partner, her interpersonal relationships — especially the quality of the relationship with her sexual partner, other psychosocial stresses (including her attitudes to middle-age, menopause and hysterectomy where relevant), any psychiatric or organic contributing factors including hormonal status as indicated by the presence of associated symptoms of hormone deficiency such as hot flushes or atrophic vaginal changes and investigation of endocrinological parameters. Chakravarti et al (1979) showed that women with sexual complaints at the menopause were more likely to respond to oestrogen therapy if plasma FSH was gretater than 15 U/l and vasomotor symptoms were present.

An integrated approach to management is needed which will aim at reducing contributory hormonal, psychological and social stress and promoting a positive adaptation to this developmental phase. This management approach has been detailed in the text *Gynaecology, Sex and Psyche* (Dennerstein et al, 1978b). Interventions which may be helpful include:

Hormonal. Where there is evidence of ovarian deficiency, oestrogen administration will reduce any biological vulnerability. When prescribing oestrogen the advantages must be balanced against the risks for any individual woman. A progestogen must be administered for the last seven to ten days of the cycle where the uterus is still intact. Whilst great benefits have been claimed for the addition of an androgen to such hormone replacement therapy, adequate evaluation of the effects of androgens has not been carried out.

Cognitive psychotherapy. Therapy sessions are orientated towards providing the woman with a more positive view of herself and her own sexuality, and of menopause and hysterectomy where appropriate. These viewpoints may be reinforced with suitable references for patients such as the book by Dennerstein, Wood and Burrows (1982). Individual sessions with the woman are often needed to explore her attitudes and facilitate a change. Conjoint sessions with both partners increase knowledge and awareness of sexuality. In particular, reference is needed to aging changes in sexuality affecting both the male and female, such as the increased time needed for arousal and the necessity for more direct stimulation of the genital areas. Conjoint sessions aim also at improving the couple's communication about sexuality and increasing their understanding of each other.

Structured behavioural tasks. These may be individually directed, as for example in helping a woman to increase her acceptance of her own body by encouraging self-examination. The most frequently used couple-directed behavioural intervention programme is the use of sensate focus or pleasuring exercises. These were developed by Masters and Johnson (1970) and aim at reducing performance-type sexual anxiety by placing a moratorium on sexual intercourse. The couple is then instructed in a series of pleasuring exercises aimed at increasing use of arousal techniques whilst facilitating the sexual communication of the couple. The successful use of this technique depends on the presence of a stable, caring relationship with both partners motivated for therapy. Where there are longstanding and more deeply-seated conflicts about sexuality a more intensive psychotherapy may be needed. Marital counselling techniques are more appropriate where interpersonal conflict is present.

CONCLUSIONS

In this review we sought evidence to determine whether changes in sexual behaviour could be expected with hormone depletion at the menopause and the effects of hormone replacement therapy on sexual response. Pronounced changes were found in female animals with oophorectomy. In primates normal sexual behaviour could be restored with administration of oestradiol and progesterone in doses approximating plasma levels of hormones during the menstrual cycle. In humans bilateral oophorectomy is usually performed in conjunction with hysterectomy, making it difficult to assess the effects of hormone depletion alone. Epidemiological studies suggest a decline in female sexual interest, orgasm and coital frequency at the menopause. There have been few double-blind studies of the effects of hormone replacement therapy on sexuality. Our own studies suggest that oestrogen does have a stimulatory effect on sexual interest, vaginal lubrication, enjoyment and orgasmic frequency in oophorectomized women. The effects of androgens in menopausal women have not been adequately evaluated. As the menopause involves biological, psychological and social stresses the therapy approach to women with sexual dysfunction at the menopause should involve consideration of all these factors. The administration of specific hormone replacement therapy may reduce any biological vulnerability. The use of other interventions, such as marital and family counselling and sex therapy techniques, are usually needed to effect a positive change when sexual problems present in association with the menopause.

REFERENCES

Asch, R. H. & Greenblatt, R. (1977) Steroidogenesis in the postmenopausal ovary. *Clinical Obstetrics and Gynecology*, **4**, 85.

Bart, P. B. & Grossman, M. (1978) Menopause in the woman patient. In *Sexual and Reproductive Aspects of Women's Health Care*. Volume **1**, pp. 337-354. New York: Plenum Press.

Benedek, T. (1950) Climacterium: a development phase. *Psychoanalytic Quarterly*, **19**, 1-27.

Bullock, J. L., Massey, F. M. & Gambrell, R. D. (1975) Use of medroxyprogesterone acetate to prevent menopausal symptoms. *Obstetrics and Gynecology*, **46**, 165-168.

Campbell, S. (1976) Double blind psychometric studies on the effects of natural estrogens on post-menopausal women. In *The Management of the Menopause and Post-Menopausal Years* (Ed.) Campbell, S. pp. 149-158. Lancaster: MTP Press.

Chakravarti, S., Collins, W. P., Newton, J. R., Oram, D. H. & Studd, J. W. (1977) Endocrine changes and symptomatology after oophorectomy in premenopausal women. *British Journal of Obstetrics and Gynecology*, **84**, 767.

Chakravarti, S., Collins, W. P., Thom, M. H. & Studd, J. W. W. (1979) Relation between plasma hormone profiles, symptoms and response to oestrogen treatment in women approaching the menopause. *British Medical Journal*, **i**, 983-985.

Crawford, M. P. & Hooper, D. (1975) Menopause, ageing and family. *Social Science and Medicine*, **7**, 469-482.

Cullberg, J., Gelli, M. G. & Jonssen, C. (1969) Mental and sexual adjustment before and after six months use of an oral contraceptive. *Acta Psychiatrica Scandinavica*, **45**, 259-276.

Davidson, J. M. (1972) Hormones and reproductive behaviour. In *Hormones and Behaviour* (Ed.) Levine, S. pp. 63-103. London: Academic Press.

Dennerstein, L., Wood, C. & Burrows, G. D. (1977) Sexual response following hysterectomy and oophorectomy. *Obstetrics and Gynecology*, **49**, 92-96.

Dennerstein, L., Wood, C. & Burrows, G. D. (1982) *Hysterectomy: How to Deal with the Physical and Emotional Aspects*. Melbourne: Oxford University Press.

Dennerstein, L., Burrows, G. D., Senior, J. & Wood, C. (1978a) Hormone replacement therapy at the menopause — a double blind controlled study of women's preferences. *Australian and New Zealand Journal of Obstetrics and Gynecology,* **18,** 139-143.

Dennerstein, L., Burrows, G. D., Cox, L. & Wood, C. (1978a) *Gynaecology, Sex and Psyche*. University Press Melbourne.

Dennerstein, L., Burrows, G. D., Wood, C. & Hyman, G. (1980) Hormones and sexuality: effect of oestrogen and progestogen. *Obstetrics and Gynecology,* **56,** 316-322.

Deutsch, H. (1945) The psychology of women. *Motherhood*. Volume 2. pp. 456-485. New York: Grune and Stratton.

Dmowski, W. P., Luna, M. & Scommegna, A. (1974) Hormonal aspects of female sexual response. *Medical Aspects of Human Sexuality,* **8,** 92-113.

Dodds, D. T., Potgieter, C. R., Turner, P. J. et al. (1961) The physical and emotional results of hysterectomy: a review of 162 cases. *South African Medical Journal,* **35,** 53-54.

Drellich, M. G. & Bieber, I. (1958) The psychological importance of the uterus and its functions. *Journal of Nervous Disorders,* **126,** 322-336.

Ellison, R. M. (1964) Psychiatric complications following sterilisation of women. *Medical Journal of Australia,* **2,** 625-628.

Everitt, B. J. (1977) Cerebral monoamines and sexual behaviour. In *Handbook of Sexology* (Ed.) Money, J. & Musaph, H. pp. 429-448. Elsevier/North Holland Biomedical Press.

Feder, H. H. (1977) Regulation of sexual behaviour by hormones in female nonprimates. In *Handbook of Sexology* (Ed.) Money, J. & Musaph, H. pp. 395-411. Elsevier/North-Holland Biomedical Press.

Fedor-Freybergh, P. (1977) The influence of oestrogens on the wellbeing and mental performance in climacteric and postmenopausal women. *Acta Obstetrica et Gynecologica Scandinavica* (Supplement 64).

Flint, M. (1975) The menopause: reward or punishment? *Psychosomatics,* **16,** 161-163.

Freud, S. (1905) Three essays on the theory of sexuality. In *The Standard Edition of the Complete Psychological Works of Sigmund Freud* ·(Ed.) Strachey, J., Freud, A., Strachey, A. & Tyson, A. Volume VII. pp. 135-243. London, The Hogarth Press and the Institute of Psychoanalysis (1968).

Gath, D., Cooper, P. & Day, A. (1982) Hysterectomy and psychiatric disorder: levels of psychiatric morbidity before and after hysterectomy. *British Journal of Psychiatry* (in press).

Hällström, T. (1977) Sexuality in the climacteric. In *Clinics in Obstetrics and Gynaecology: The Menopause,* **4,** 227-239. (Ed.) Greenblatt, R. B. & Studd, J. Eastbourne: W. B. Saunders.

Herbert, J. (1977) The neuroendocrine basis of sexual behaviour in primates. In *Handbook of Sexology* (Ed.) Money, J. & Musaph, H. pp. 449-459. Elsevier/North-Holland Biomedical Press.

Huffman, J. W. (1950) The effect of gynecologic surgery on sexual reactions. *American Journal of Obstetrics and Gynecology,* **59,** 915-917.

Kamberi, I. A. & Kobayashi, Y. (1970) Monoamine oxidase activity in the hypothalamus and various other brain areas and in some endocrine glands of the rat during the oestrus cycle. *Journal of Neurochemistry,* **17,** 261-268.

Keverne, E. B. (1977) Pheromones and sexual behaviour. In *Handbook of Sexology* (Ed.) Money, J. & Musaph, H. pp. 413-428. Elsevier/North-Holland Biomedical Press.

Kinsey, A. C., Pomeroy, W. B., Martin, C. E. & Gebhard, P. H. (1953) *Sexual Behaviour in the Human Female*. Philadelphia: Saunders.

Krystal, S. & Chiriboga, D. A. (1979) The empty nest process in mid-life men and women. *Maturitas,* **1,** 215-222.

Lauritzen, C. (1973) The Management of the premenopausal and the postmenopausal patient. In *Ageing and Estrogens* (Ed.) Van Keep, P. A. & Lauritzen, C. pp. 2-21. Basel: Karger.

Martin, R. L., Roberts, W. V. & Clayton, P. J. (1980) Psychiatric status after hysterectomy. *Journal of the American Medical Association,* **244,** 350-353.

Masters, W. H. & Johnson, V. E. (1966) *Human Sexual Response*. Boston: Little Brown.

Masters, W. H. & Johnson, V. E. (1970) *Human Sexual Inadequacy*. Boston: Little Brown.

Michael, R. P. & Bonsall, R. W. (1977) Peri-ovulatory synchronisation of behaviour in male and female rhesus monkeys. *Nature,* **265,** 463-464.

Michael, R. P., Keverne, E. B. & Bonsall, R. W. (1971) Pheromones: isolation of male sex attractants from a female primate. *Science,* **172,** 964-966.

Munday, R. N. & Cox, L. W. (1967) Hysterectomy for benign lesions. *Medical Journal of Australia,* **2,** 759-763.

Naftolin, F., Ryan, K. J., Davies, I. J. et al. (1975) The formation of estrogens by central neuroendocrine tissues. *Recent Progress in Hormone Research,* **31,** 295-319.

Patterson, R. M. & Craig, J. B. (1963) Misconceptions concerning the psychological effects of hysterectomy. *American Journal of Obstetrics & Gynecology,* **85,** 104-111.

Pfeiffer, E., Verwoerdt, A. & Davis, G. C. (1972) Sexual behaviour in middle life. *American Journal of Psychiatry,* **128,** 1262-1267.

Ricci, J. V. (1943) *The Genealogy of Gynaecology.* Philadelphia: Blakiston.

Richards, D. H. (1974) A post-hysterectomy syndrome. *Lancet,* **ii,** 983-985.

Schneider, M. & Brotherton, P. (1979) Physiological, psychological and situational stresses in depression during the climacteric. *Maturitas,* **1,** 153-158.

Smith, D. C., Prentice, R. & Thompson, D. J. (1975) Association of exogenous estrogen and endometrial carcinoma. *New England Journal of Medicine,* **293,** 1164-1167.

Studd, J., Chakravarti, S. & Oram, D. (1977) The climacteric. In *Clinics in Obstetrics and Gynaecology: The Menopause,* **4,** 3-29. (Ed.) Greenblatt, R. B. & Studd, J. Eastbourne: W. B. Saunders.

Utian, W. H. (1972) The true clinical features of post-menopause and oophorectomy and their response to oestrogen therapy. *South African Medical Journal,* **46,** 732-737.

Utian, W. H. (1975) Effect of hysterectomy, oophorectomy and estrogen therapy on libido. *International Journal of Obstetrics and Gynaecology,* **13,** 97-100.

van Keep, P. A. & Kellerhals, J. M. (1974) The impact of sociocultural factors on symptom formation. *Psychotherapy and Psychomatics,* **23,** 251-263.

Whalen, R. E. (1966) Sexual motivation. *Psychological Review,* **73,** 151-163.

Ziel, H. K. & Finkle, W. D. (1975) Increased risk of endometrial carcinoma among users of conjugated estrogens. *New England Journal of Medicine,* **293,** 1167-1170.

Zussman, L., Zussman, S., Sunley, R. & Bjornson, E. (1981) Sexual response after hysterectomy-oophorectomy: recent studies and reconsideration of psychogenesis. *American Journal of Obstetrics and Gynecology,* **140,** 725-729.

5

Hormones and Psychosexual Differentiation: Implications for the Management of Intersexuality, Homosexuality and Transsexuality

HEINO F. L. MEYER-BAHLBURG

INTRODUCTION

For the endocrinologist, one of the most difficult clinical tasks is the management of patients with intersexuality and gender identity disorders requiring decisions on sex of assignment or sex reassignment; not only are the diagnostic assessment procedures complex, but also the decisions involve emotionally highly-charged value judgments. Furthermore, comprehensive patient care in this area requires the cooperation of several disciplines, as does the research that provides the theoretical background for the clinical decisions.

Over the last decade, both the biological and the social sciences have made major advances in elucidating the basic foundations of psychosexual differentiation. The *Clinics* are not the place to give a comprehensive overview of these developments, especially since there is a new series of concise review papers that are easily accessible to most clinicians (Naftolin and Butz, 1981; see also Lewis and Weinraub, 1979). Instead, I will briefly sketch current conceptual issues and recent empirical data from psychoendocrine research that are of direct relevance to clinical decision-making.

Clinically, the most important categories of sex-dimorphic behaviour that need to be considered in this context are (1) *gender identity*, that is, the primary identification of an individual with one sex or the other; (2) *gender-role behaviour*, which refers to those aspects of behaviour in which normal males and females differ in a given culture, for instance, social play (rough-and-tumble or not), sex preferences in peer association, parenting rehearsal, social aggression, sexual behaviour, etc.; (3) *sexual orientation*, or the degree of erotic responsiveness to one sex or the other, as assessed by imagery, attractions, and, secondarily, overt behaviour. Except for gender identity, which presupposes language development, all categories of human sex-dimorphic behaviour mentioned have their parallels in animal behaviour.

Clinics in Endocrinology and Metabolism — Vol. 11, No. 3, November 1982.
0300-595X/82/11.03/681 $03.00 © 1982 W. B. Saunders Company Ltd

In lower mammals, sex-dimorphic behaviour is regulated by brain systems that are differentiated or *organized* during hormone-sensitive periods early in development, that is, pre- or perinatally (MacLusky and Naftolin, 1981). Central nervous system organization for masculine behaviour will ensue if sufficient androgens are available during this sensitive period, and feminine or intermediate behaviour will result if androgens are deficient or if the enzymes and/or receptors necessary for androgen utilization are lacking. These early effects of hormones are independent of chromosomal or gonadal status of the individual. That we deal here with genuine organizational effects is proved by the demonstration of structural changes induced by androgen, such as variations in the size of certain cell nuclei, in dendritic growth, or in synaptic organization (Toran-Allerand, 1980; MacLusky and Naftolin, 1981). The main areas of the brain involved in this differentiation process are the hypothalamus, the preoptic area, and the amygdala. The brain systems underlying sex-dimorphic behaviour are in close proximity to those involved in gonadotrophin regulation; the organization of the latter also depends on androgens. Therefore, in lower mammals, the differentiation of the gonadotrophin regulation as cyclic (in normal females) and tonic (in normal males) usually runs in parallel with the differentiation of sex-dimorphic behaviour.

To some extent the sex hormone-dependent structural organization of the brain parallels the differentiation of the external genitalia; also, in the latter case, males and females start with the same anlagen which then differentiate as male or female, depending on the presence or absence of systemic androgen (Wilson, George and Griffin, 1981). However, there are important differences in the biochemical mechanisms involved. For instance, the fetal differentiation of the external genitalia depends on dihydrotestosterone, the 5-alpha-reduced metabolite of testosterone. By contrast, in a number of species, fetal brain effects of sex hormones seem to depend, at least in part, on aromatization of testosterone to oestradiol (Bardin and Catterall, 1981; McEwen, 1981). There are also differences in timing, with the differentiation of the genitalia preceding the sex-dimorphic differentiation of the brain. Such findings are important because they point the way to possible explanations of discrepancies between body and brain development, similar to the way discrepancies in the development of internal and external genitalia can be explained by various specific enzyme or hormone abnormalities.

Postnatally, some categories of sex-dimorphic behaviour, for instance social play in childhood, apparently unfold without specific hormonal prompting. Others, such as mating behaviour, are *activated* by the increasing levels of sex hormones in puberty (Rubin, Reinisch and Haskett, 1981).

In subhuman primates the available data are much more scanty, yet seem to parallel the findings in lower mammals except for a stronger contribution of social factors to the development of sex-dimorphic behaviour.

Whether and to what extent sex differences in the behaviour of human beings can be attributed to prenatal hormone conditions is currently a matter of intense debate. Certainly, the biological prerequisites are given.

One is the comparability of the hypothalamic and adjacent brain systems across mammalian species. Another is the existence of fetal sex differences in hormonal levels throughout most of pregnancy (Forest, de Peretti and Bertrand, 1980), including the period of hypothalamic differentiation (in man, presumably the second trimester of pregnancy: Dörner and Staudt, 1972). Some of the available evidence supporting an influence of prenatal hormones on human psychosexual differentiation will be cited below.

INTERSEXUALITY

The classical approach to sex assignment of patients with ambiguous genitalia has been to determine the 'prevailing' somatic sex by examining the gonads, including their histology (or more recently the karyotype). If the diagnosis had been made correctly, a gender-appropriate development was expected. However, over the years cases came to light that did not seem to follow such a simple principle. Already Ellis (1945) had concluded from a review of 84 published cases that the gender identity ('sex role') of a hermaphrodite 'accords primarily not with his or her internal and external somatic characteristics, but rather with his or her masculine or feminine upbringing'. Yet it was the work by Money and the Hampsons at Johns Hopkins that led to a major change in the traditional policy. In their papers of 1955 (a, b) and 1956 they summarized their own rich case material and formulated a new criterion for the sex assignment of intersex patients, namely, the expected future social and, especially, sexual functioning.

The proposal of Money and the Hampsons was based on two major conclusions from their data on 76 intersexed patients: (1) Gender identity *can* develop independently of and in contrast to gonadal histology, karyotype, internal genitals, even external genitals and secondary sexual characteristics, singly or in combination. 'The evidence of hermaphroditism lends support to a conception that, psychologically, sexuality is undifferentiated at birth and that it becomes differentiated as masculine or feminine in the course of the various experiences of growing up' (Money, Hampson and Hampson, 1955b, p. 308). The best 'prognosticator' of gender identity is the sex of assignment and rearing (Money, Hampson and Hampson, 1955b, p. 319). (2) The development of gender identity and gender role behaviour is similar to imprinting (and can be compared to early language acquisition), beginning at 12 months, reaching a critical period at 18 months, and being relatively well-established by two and a half years (Money, Hampson and Hampson, 1955b, pp. 309-310). Although the authors asserted that 'gender role may be changed' at a later age (Money, Hampson and Hampson, 1955b, p. 310), they presented data showing increasing risk of psychopathology with increasing age at the time of reassignment (Money, Hampson and Hampson, 1956). Ambiguity of gender identity was identified as a consequence of ambiguity of rearing, and medical management was directed to minimize this risk: by speeding up diagnostic procedures, by providing intense medical education and counselling to the parents so that they could become active participants in the decision process, and by surgically correcting the appearance of the external genitals in concordance with the assigned sex before the infant left the hospital (Money, 1968, 1975). With the weight of Lawson Wilkins' and later Robert Blizzard's paediatric endocrinology at Johns Hopkins Hospital behind it, sex of assignment on the basis of future social and sexual functioning became a widely adopted policy.

One particular aspect of the original approach by Money and the Hampsons, namely, the assumption of an 'undifferentiated' sexuality at birth, was dropped when subsequent research demonstrated that prenatal hormones influence certain aspects of human sex-dimorphic behaviour in the same direction as that of other mammals. The evidence came from behavioural studies of patients with prenatal endocrine syndromes or a history of maternal hormone treatment during pregnancy. A number of researchers, especially Ehrhardt, Money and their colleagues, provided pertinent data. These have been extensively reviewed in Money and Ehrhardt (1972) and updated in Ehrhardt and Meyer-Bahlburg (1981). The overall conclusion is that prenatal hormones specifically affect gender-role behaviour. For instance, girls exposed to high levels of androgen in fetal life as a result of either maternal drug treatment or of congenital adrenal hyperplasia were found to show markedly increased rough-and-tumble play, decreased parenting rehearsal, etc. Typically, such shifts in sex-dimorphic behaviour could be accommodated within the range of behaviour accepted for a given gender, since normal males and females show wide variations and much overlap in gender-role behaviour. Thus gender identity usually agreed with the sex of assignment and rearing unless the latter had been ambiguous. Here then was a demonstration that gender identity can develop and be maintained even in contrast to what presumably are direct effects of hormones on the brain — further support for the management policy of Money, Hampson and Hampson (1955a).

More recently, however, this position has been questioned on the basis of the newly-diagnosed syndrome of 5-alpha-reductase deficiency by Imperato-McGinley and coworkers (1974, 1979). Its developmental course frequently seems to involve a reversal of gender identity in adolescence which has led to a view radically different from Money's: '. . . it appears that the extent of androgen (i.e., testosterone) exposure of the brain in utero, during the early postnatal period and at puberty has more effect in determining male-gender identity than does sex of rearing. This experiment of nature emphasizes the importance of androgens, which act as inducers (in utero and neonatally) and as activators (at puberty), in the evolution of a male-gender identity' (Imperato-McGinley et al, 1979). Thus, direct CNS mediation of hormonal effects on gender identity is postulated. This new theory has led to a marked insecurity on the part of those who have to make decisions on sex assignment and reassignment. I will therefore review the evidence in some detail.

Male pseudohermaphrodites with 5-alpha-reductase deficiency suffer from impaired metabolism of testosterone to dihydrotestosterone which results in severe ambiguity of the external genitalia (Imperato-McGinley et al, 1979). These patients are born with a markedly bifid scrotum that appears labia-like, a clitoris-like phallus, a urogenital sinus with a blind-ending vaginal pouch, and, frequently, undescended testes. Thus, at birth, many affected infants are thought to be girls and are raised accordingly. These patients start virilizing, however, during puberty, under the influence of their own normal plasma testosterone levels. The voice deepens, and their muscles develop. There is substantial penile growth and the usual scrotal development. In most subjects, the testes descend into the scrotum. The subjects experience erections, and there is an ejaculate from the urethral orifice on the perineum. In coitus, they are capable of intromission, but because of the position of the urethra, incapable of insemination.

In their 1979 paper Imperato-McGinley et al referred to 33 living male pseudohermaphrodites with 5-alpha-reductase deficiency from 23 interrelated families spanning four generations in three rural villages of the Dominican Republic. Interview data showed that 19 of the 33 subjects had been unambiguously raised as girls. Postpubertal psychosexual data were obtained from 18 of these 19 subjects. Of the 18 subjects, 17 had changed to male gender identity and 16 to a male gender role.

In examining the available evidence, we need to answer several questions.

(1) Were the individuals who changed really brought up unambiguously as females, and did they have an unambiguous female gender identity during childhood? The authors describe the gender-typical socialization pattern for normal children in this particular society but do not give specific information on their patients' upbringing, probably due to the fact that most of them were seen only in late adolescence or adulthood. Since the condition became quite well-known in the area, there seems to have been a change in rearing practices; currently many of these children are recognized early and reared as boys. This observation indicates that the villagers themselves can recognize the ambiguity of the genitalia in many of these children, and it raises the question whether that might have been the case already in some of the older patients. It is clear from the reports and the published photographs (Peterson et al, 1977) that in infancy and childhood the genital appearance of the affected individuals is definitely not masculine. Yet the enlarged clitoris, the urogenital sinus and the partial labial fusion are not identical with normal female genitalia which may have led to gender doubts and ambiguous rearing by at least some of the family members. Moreover, the authors do not provide developmental data on the behavioural and temperamental characteristics of these individuals nor on their gender identity during childhood.

(2) As adults, did these patients really have a full male-gender identity? Among the 18 documented patients, there were two exceptions: one subject changed to a male-gender identity but continued to dress as a woman; the other maintained a female gender identity and role and desired corrective surgery of her genitalia. The other 16 dressed, worked, and had sexual or marital relationships with women like normal men, and 'were convinced that they were men'. Thus, apart from the two exceptions, it seems that most of these subjects really lived as men, yet the definitive establishment of a fully male-gender identity requires more detailed interview data. The conclusion is that the published accounts do not permit us to decide whether or not there was a genuine change of gender identity from childhood to

adulthood. However, Imperato-McGinley and colleagues are not the only researchers to report gender identity changes in adolescence. For instance, Gajdusek (1977) has described a similar phenomenon in tribal societies of New Guinea. Wolf (1968) has reviewed such cases in the Western literature, and further case studies have been published since then. The majority of reports on gender identity changes concern male pseudohermaphrodites who have been reared female, but virilize in puberty and then change their gender identity. Quite a few patients that do not change have also been noted. By and large, the quality of the available clinical reports is very variable and rarely satisfactory. Documentation of early rearing conditions, gender role behaviour, and gender identity of the patient is usually quite limited, mostly based on recall in adolescence or adulthood, and certainly does not constitute particularly reliable information. Nevertheless, on the basis of the published reports and of my own experience with patients who developed gender identity disorders after an apparently unambiguous gender identity had been established, I think it is likely that there are quite a few individuals who have genuinely changed their childhood gender identity in adolescence or later, and I question not so much the phenomenon of change itself as the mechanism proposed.

(3) Does the evidence support a neuroendocrine basis for gender identity development? Imperato-McGinley et al postulate a hormone effect on the brain as the primary mechanism of gender-identity development. However, in distinction from other sex-dimorphic behaviours, there is no phenomenon in animals that corresponds to gender identity, and a hormone-dependent sex-dimorphic neural substrate for this language-related function is hard to imagine. Also, the timing of the change process is unusual: the 17 subjects who changed '. . . began to realize that they were different from other girls in the village between 7 and 12 years of age, when they did *not* develop breasts, when their bodies began to change in a *masculine* direction, and when masses were noted in the inguinal canal or scrotum . . . a male gender identity gradually evolved over several years as the subjects passed through stages of no longer feeling like girls, to feeling like men, and finally to the conscious awareness that they were indeed men. The change to a male-gender role occurred either during puberty or in the post-pubertal period after the subjects were convinced that they were men (male-gender identity) and were experiencing sexual interest in women. The gender-role change took place at 16 years of age, on the average, with a range of 14 to 24 years.' (Imperato-McGinley et al, 1979, p. 1234). For a primary 'activating' effect of hormones on brain, this seems to be an extraordinarily long period if compared to the effects of steroid hormones on gonadotrophin regulation or on sexual function and motivation. No similarly slow activational process is known in psychoneuroendocrinology.

I think that a combination of experiential and rational factors explains the gender identity change better than a neuroendocrine mechanism. Compared to their pubertal female peers, these patients experience a progressive decline of their physical femininity, becoming increasingly unattractive, with no capacity for vaginal intercourse, little hope for a mate, and faced with the prospect of permanent childlessness which makes for tremendous social and economic consequences in most underdeveloped agricultural societies. Certainly, the reactions of the social environment would reflect the gender-discrepant physique. At the same time, however, the potential of these patients for a life as a male rapidly improves — along with the development of an attractive male physique, with adequate gain in muscular strength to engage in strenuous physical work, an increasingly functional male genital and testicular descent offering some (at least remote) hope for fertility, an important issue for many individuals with gender disorders. Moreover, when these patients come to medical attention, it is highly probable that their 'biological maleness' will be explained to them. Whether their sexual orientation to women plays a key role in their re-identification process, as Wolf (1968) concludes for intersexes in general, cannot be decided since we have hardly any detailed data on the sequence of events.

A purely neuroendocrine theory would also have difficulties in explaining why late-treated women with congenital adrenal hyperplasia, with both pre- and postnatal exposure to androgen and heavy virilization throughout childhood and adolescence, did not become transsexual. After medical exploration, they probably were aware of the fact that they had a uterus, ovaries, and hope for fertility which made the maintenance of their child-hood gender identity as female desirable.

Taken together, these various considerations let me reject the notion that the gender identity change of the Santo Domingo patients is primarily the result of direct effects of hormones on the brain. The process description by Imperato-McGinley et al (1979) as quoted above is much more in line with an experiential-cognitive explanation than with a neuroendocrine rationale. Certainly, the hormones play a role, but this is mediated by physical appearance, perceived functional capacities, and reactions by the social environment rather than directly by hormone-sensitive CNS systems.

In my opinion the reports on the 5-alpha-reductase deficiency syndrome do not indicate a need for a basic revision of the Hopkins policy of sex assignment and reassignment of intersex patients. What does this conclusion imply for the management of newborn males with 5-alpha-reductase deficiency or similar male pseudohermaphrodites? Should they be raised (1) female, or (2) male, or (3) first female with a planned gender change at puberty? First of all, the principle remains that the decision on sex assignment must be made early after birth and should remain final unless the patient him- or herself desires change later. All three options listed have their problems. The third one impresses me as the most unrealistic because unambiguous rearing of the female seems nearly impossible when the parents know about the child's condition, and because gender identity cannot be changed by prescription. To live in our society as a male with no male genitals in childhood and with only a half-sized penis plus a perineal urethral meatus in adulthood, which is the implication of option (2), is likely to make a successful social and sexual performance of the male role very difficult. Thus, sex assignment as female with early medical inter-vention and complete prevention of or immediate interference with pubertal virilization appears to present the smallest risk.

Male pseudohermaphrodites reared as girls who are referred to our Psychoendocrine Clinic early in adolescence because of pubertal virilization are typically bothered by these somatic changes which are incongruent with their gender identity. They want medical corrections, and our detailed interview work-ups do not indicate gender dysphoria. Once the appropriate surgical and hormonal corrections are performed, their further development progresses along female lines (e.g., Ehrhardt, 1979). Whether with uninhibited progressive virilization and accompanying alienation from the normal developmental path of their peer group these patients may develop gender dysphoria and finally decide for gender identity change is hard to predict; at the very least, such a course of events implies a major stress with unpredictable psychiatric consequences, a risk which I am unprepared to recommend.

HOMOSEXUALITY

In 1973 the American Psychiatric Association decided that homosexuality per se does not constitute a mental disorder, and the term was removed from the subsequent revision of the Diagnostic and Statistical Manual of Psychiatric Disorders (DSM-III). A residual category, 'Ego-dystonic Homosexuality', remained, 'reserved for those homosexuals for whom changing sexual orientation is a *persistent* concern.' Regardless of this distinction, parents or relatives of homosexuals often ask physicians whether hormones play a part in homosexuality and if so whether there is some form of hormonal treatment available. Therefore, I will briefly review the current status of the psychoendocrinology of sexual orientation. (For a detailed presentation of data and conceptual issues see Meyer-Bahlburg, 1977, 1979).

Homo- and heterosexual orientation as used here refers to the degree of sexual responsiveness to the same and/or other sex, expressed in erotic attractions, sexual fantasies, and (not necessarily) actual sexual experiences. By contrast, homosexual and heterosexual *behaviour* refers to any sexual act between members of the same or opposite sex, regardless of their sexual orientation. Following Kinsey, Pomeroy and Martin (1948), sexual orientation is defined operationally on a rating scale continuum ranging from 0, exclusive heterosexuality, to 6, exclusive homosexuality, with the midpoint at 3, equal sexual responsiveness to both males and females. This rating is typically based on interview material. In most psychoendocrine studies subjects from both poles are contrasted. The assessment of sexual orientation can be refined by direct measurement of genital arousal in response to sexual stimuli, that is, by penile plethysmography (e.g., Abel and Blanchard, 1976) in males or corresponding vaginal measures for females (e.g., Heiman, 1978).

From an endocrinological point of view, homosexuality is conceptualized as a problem of intersexuality. Since primary and secondary sex characteristics and sex chromosomes are typically normal in homosexual individuals, the search for indicators of intersexuality has concentrated on the sex hormones, starting with urinary hormone excretion earlier in this century and focusing on plasma hormone levels during the last decade. For males, this search has been largely negative. (For references see Meyer-Bahlburg, 1980; added to the current review were Wilson and Fulford, 1977; Futterweit, 1980; and Meyer et al, 1981). Of a total of 24 studies published since 1971, only four found lower testosterone means for homosexual than for heterosexual males, 18 studies showed no systematic difference, and two showed elevated levels of testosterone. Studies of the blood production rate of testosterone and of free or unbound testosterone gave essentially similar results. Attempts at finding hormonal differences between effeminate and non-effeminate homosexuals or between individuals that take the active or passive coital role did not lead to consistent findings. Also the data on oestrogen levels, from seven different studies, are negative or inconsistent. The lack of clinical significance of the steroid findings is underlined by the fact that the 15 studies available on gonadotrophin levels likewise present essentially negative results. In summary, it appears that sexual orientation in males is not correlated with the androgen-oestrogen balance in adolescence or adulthood.

Somewhat less clearcut is the situation in females, where only a relatively small number of reports is available. There does not seem to be a hormonal difference between the majority of adult homosexual and heterosexual women. Yet about one-third of homosexual (including gender-identity-disordered or transsexual) women examined showed somewhat elevated testosterone levels. For instance, Gartrell, Loriaux and Chase (1977) compared 21 homosexual women to 19 age-matched heterosexual controls and found that plasma testosterone levels averaged 38 per cent higher in homosexual than in heterosexual subjects. Even when there are elevated testosterone levels, they are far below the male range. We do not know whether these data constitute artefacts of sampling incurred, for instance, by the exclusion of endocrinopathies such as hirsutism or Stein-Leventhal syndrome from the normal control samples but not from the homosexual samples, or artefacts of hormone assays, caused for instance by the analysis of homo- and heterosexual subjects in separate batches or in non-blind procedures.

If the androgen findings hold up in future replications, it needs to be determined whether the elevated androgens are of ovarian or adrenal origin. In either case, elevated testosterone could be interpreted as an aetiological factor in the development of female homosexuality or as a consequence of homosexual orientation. For instance, one could follow the argument of Friedman et al (1977) that homosexuals differ from heterosexual controls in emotional stress since they belong to a repressed minority in a homophobic culture; chronic stress of this kind may lead to chronically increased activation of the pituitary adrenal axis resulting in increased output of androstenedione which then is peripherally converted to testosterone. Note, however, that such considerations would apply to only one-third of female homosexuals.

In recent years the major focus of psychoendrocrine research on sexual orientation has shifted from the hormone situation in adulthood to the role of prenatal hormones. This approach is based on the animal research described in the beginning of this chapter. It was the endocrinologist Dörner (1967, 1968, 1976) in East Berlin who most forcefully extrapolated from animal experimentation to human behaviour. He called his sex-dimorphically inverted rats 'homosexual' and introduced them as a biological model of the development of human sexual orientation. Currently, the theory enjoys tremendous attention and acceptance not only among biologists and physicians but also by behavioural scientists who are dissatisfied with the status of psychosocial explanations (e.g., Bell, Weinberg and Hammersmith, 1981) and by behaviour therapists frustrated by the low success rate of behavioural methods in changing sexual orientation in change-motivated patients (e.g., MacCulloch and Waddington, 1981; McConaghy, 1981).

The complex brain systems involved in the regulation of mating behaviour in lower mammals have largely been delineated (Pfaff, 1980). Simplifying the available data, Dörner (1976) suggested a dual mating centre theory with the medial preoptic/anterior hypothalamic region mainly involved in the regulation of male sexual behaviour (mounting, intromission, ejaculation) and the ventromedial nuclear region in the regulation of female sexual behaviour (lordosis). The differentiation of these centres is under the control of perinatal hormones. If perinatal androgens are high, they will lead to the predominant organization of the 'male centre'; if androgens are low, the 'female centre' will predominate. Predominance of the male or female centre predisposes an individual for a specific sexual orientation. If the predominant differentiation of the female centre occurs in a genetically and somatically male individual, he will be predisposed for homosexuality. If the male centre develops in a genetically and somatically female individual, she will be predisposed to homosexuality, and vice versa. Bisexuality in either sex represents the effects of intermediate levels of androgens in the fetus. In analogy to genital differentiation, Dörner (1976) categorizes homosexuality as a 'central nervous pseudohermaphroditism'.

If this theory is valid, it follows directly that a genuine causal therapy or prevention of the development of a homosexual orientation has to focus on the early differentiation phase of the brain with the aim of optimizing androgen effects on the fetus. Since the early hormonal situation leads to irreversible structural organizations in the brain, the only treatment approach later in development or in adulthood is the destruction of the overdifferentiated sex centre, and such a psychosurgical approach has already been used in the treatment of 'intractable' paedophilic homosexuality (Müller et al, 1974), although its justification and the unsatisfying documentation of its effects have been criticized (Schmidt and Schorsch, 1981).

In validating Dörner's theory for the human case, several major difficulties have arisen. One such problem is that the rat model itself is at variance with the theory. Both the rat model and the theory predict that prenatal androgen deficiency in males will lead to feminine sexual behaviour, interpreted as male homosexuality, in the presence of normal plasma testosterone levels in adulthood. In contrast to the theory, however, the rat model does not predict preferential homosexuality in gonadally intact females (which is the typical condition of the human female homosexual), since Dörner found predominant 'homosexuality' in prenatally androgenized female rats only after gonadectomy and testosterone administration in adulthood; if left gonadally intact, the rats showed just a slight increase in mounting behaviour but a very clear predominance of female sexual behaviour.

Another problem for Dörner's theory is the fact that in most animal studies of this kind, systemic manipulation of sex hormones in the pre- or perinatal stage of development results not only in shifts of sex-dimorphic behaviour and in structural changes of the underlying brain systems but also in corresponding alterations of the genitalia. By contrast, the typical human homosexual has normal gender-appropriate genitalia. Thus, we need animal models in which pre- or perinatal hormone variations lead to shifts in sex-dimorphic mating behaviour but do not affect genital development. One such model could involve the timing of prenatal events. Since in mammalian ontogenesis, genital differentiation typically predates hypothalamic differentiation, careful timing of a hormonal intervention may affect the one without the other. An alternative explanation for the lack of correlation of genital development and sexual orientation in homosexuals may lie in differences between brain and genitals in the biochemical mechanisms of androgen utilization. For instance, a defect in the brain-cell-based aromatization of testosterone to oestradiol and/or in the latter's receptor binding should lead to disturbances in male brain differentiation without affecting the genitalia. Temporary changes in hormone production and/or utilization may be induced by environmental stress. This must be implied by the findings of Ward (1972, 1977) who was able to induce lasting feminization of mating behaviour in male rats without affecting genital appearance by exposing the pregnant mother to light and heat stress during the last part of pregnancy. Based on these results, war stress affecting the pregnant mother has been suggested as an aetiological factor for homosexual men born during the 1940s (e.g., Dörner et al, 1980). Many other possible mechanisms are being considered. For instance, MacCulloch and Waddington (1981) have proposed that there may be a spontaneous generation of antibodies to testosterone by the pregnant mother of a male fetus with a consequent increase in biologically inactive serum testosterone leading to behavioural demasculinization in the fetus; they discussed a similar mechanism for female development. At this time, all these possibilities present more problems than solutions and have to await further conceptual and empirical work.

A further major difficulty for the prenatal-hormone theory of sexual orientation arises from the study of endocrine syndromes with known prenatal hormone abnormalities. The available evidence, mainly based on studies by Money, Ehrhardt and coworkers (for references see Meyer-Bahlburg, 1977, 1979), appears to indicate an overriding influence of the sex of assignment and rearing and of the resulting gender identity on sexual orientation. For instance, the majority of early treated genetically female patients with congenital adrenal hyperplasia (CAH) were found to be heterosexual; it is not known whether the low frequency of bisexual or homosexual individuals observed is increased above that in unselected women without CAH since no adequate control groups were used. Even in the most extreme patient group, however, that is late-treated CAH women with both pre- and postnatal virilization, homosexuals did not predominate (Ehrhardt, Evers and Money, 1968). The findings in genetic male pseudo-hermaphrodites appear similar. Genetic males that have been assigned to the female sex in early childhood yet develop a sexual orientation towards females in adolescence typically seem either to come from a background of ambiguous rearing and/or to develop their discrepant sexual orientation under the influence of gender-discrepant puberty, thus in a quite different situation than the typical non-intersexed homosexual.

Do homosexuals show any functional characteristics that could indicate prenatal hormone abnormalities? The positive oestrogen feedback effect on luteinizing hormone (LH) has been suggested as such an indicator. This phenomenon is well established for females where oestrogen levels rise in the follicular phase of the menstrual cycle and elicit an LH surge which triggers ovulation. The same effect can be achieved by administration of oestrogens. In males, however, the effect is much harder to achieve. The oestrous cycle of the normal female rat shows a very similar phenomenon. The LH response to oestrogen cannot be elicited, however, when the rats have been neonatally androgenized. Dörner (1976) argued that homosexual men should show a stronger positive feedback effect than heterosexual men if male homosexuality is in fact due to a deficiency of prenatal andro-genization of the brain. His research group has presented data showing the expected differences between male homosexuals and heterosexuals (Dörner, 1976). Corresponding data for female transsexuals (with homosexual orientation) were presented by Dörner et al (1976) and Seyler et al (1978). These findings are in urgent need of replication by independent laboratories. Regulation of LH is a complicated phenomenon involving both negative and positive feedback mechanisms. In contrast to lower mammals, the gonadotrophin regulation of non-human primates shows only little influence of prenatal hormones (Karsch, Dierschke and Knobil, 1973; Steiner et al, 1976) and depends largely on current sex hormone levels in adolescence and adulthood. Thus minor variations of endogenous steroid levels in the circulation as well as hormone intake, as practised by trans-sexuals, are likely to affect gonadotrophin regulation. Also, LH dynamics do not necessarily parallel sexual orientation. For instance, two recent studies of gonadally intact genetic males with the complete syndrome of androgen insensitivity have shown that the LH response to oestrogen in the syndrome is *not* female-like but male-like, that is, after oestrogen priming, LH is suppressed rather than increased (Van Look et al, 1977; Aono et al, 1978). These patients are typically female identified and have a female heterosexual orientation in contrast to their male-like LH dynamics.

In summary, the prenatal hormone theory of sexual orientation in humans is by no means well established, but presents a major challenge to conceptualization and empirical research. The enthusiastic adherents of the prenatal hormone theory must not only come up with more decisive data that demonstrate the contribution of prenatal hormones to the development of sexual orientation in humans, they must also find an empirically validated explanation for the missing association of homosexual orientation with findings of intersex genitalia. Finally, they need to provide an explanation as to why the development of a sexual orientation as homo- or heterosexual should categorically differ from the development of such phenomena as paedophilia, fetishism, and other paraphilias for which we do not assume a hormonal basis. Those, on the other hand, who like to dismiss the psychoendocrine approach altogether must give a well-founded explanation for how human beings can totally step out of line with their mammalian ancestors — even though the critical brain structures under examination, as well as the prenatal endocrine development, are very similar to those in other mammals, and in spite of the fact that prenatal hormonal effects have already been demonstrated for other categories of sex-dimorphic behaviour in humans.

The conclusions for the practising clinician are that the current status of research does not provide a scientific basis for endocrine intervention, even in ego-dystonic homosexuals seeking treatment. If any form of inter-sexuality has been ruled out by physical examination, no additional endocrine workup, and especially no hormonal measures, are clinically justified. Inquiring patients, relatives and teachers need to be apprised of the current status of psychoendocrine research in ways appropriate to their level of education.

TRANSSEXUALITY

Gender identity disorders are characterized by an incongruence between (normal) anatomical sex and gender identity. The specific diagnosis of transsexuality applies to adolescents and adults with gender identity disorder who wish to be rid of their own genitalia and to live as a member of the other sex, and in whom the disturbance has been continuous (not limited to periods of stress) for at least two years. These diagnostic categories of DSM-III exclude physical or chromosomal intersexuality and gender identity disorder secondary to another mental disorder such as schizophrenia.

The biological approach to the aetiology of gender identity disorders is the same as the approach to homosexuality, that is, it derives from the concept of intersexuality. In fact, in reviewing the endocrine research on sexual orientation I have combined studies on homosexual and transsexual individuals. The justification for such a combination is that we have only one comprehensive biological theory of the sexual differentiation of brain and behaviour. There is also an ontogenetic overlap between homosexual and transsexual individuals: gender identity disorder of childhood to varying degrees is a rather common finding in recall studies of both adult homosexuals (Saghir and Robins, 1973; Bell, Weinberg and Hammersmith, 1981) and transsexuals (Green, 1974), and in prospective studies gender identity disorder of childhood in males has been found to increase the likelihood of the development of transsexuality, transvestism, and/or (effeminate) homosexuality in adolescence and adulthood (Lebovitz, 1972; Zuger, 1978; Green, 1979; Money and Russo, 1979).

If one separates out the rather modest number of endocrine studies on transsexual individuals from those on non-transsexual homosexuals, the findings remain the same: there are no significant differences in sex hormone levels between the majority of transsexual individuals and heterosexual controls in both sexes, but there are somewhat increased levels of testosterone in about a third of female transsexuals. The prenatal hormone theory has been applied to transsexual individuals in the same way as to homosexual individuals, and the conceptual and empirical problems and difficulties apply as well. Recently, chromosome studies have been done on children with gender identity disorder (Green, 1976; Rekers et al, 1979); their karyotypes turned out to be normal.

A new aetiological theory of transsexuality involves the histocompatibility-Y (H-Y) antigen. H-Y antigen is a cell-surface component that is usually associated with all male tissues and appears to be directly involved in the induction of testicular differentiation (Haseltine and Ohno, 1981). Eicher and co-workers from Munich (Eicher et al, 1979; Spoljar et al, 1981) examined H-Y antigen in male and female transsexuals, compared with heterosexual controls; in the majority of cases the transsexuals had an H-Y antigen status concordant with the desired sex and discordant with the anatomical sex. A second, independent, group (Engel, Pfäfflin and Wiedeking, 1980) used a different assay and obtained similar results with regard to transsexuals, but their control group results also differed from what was expected. The measurement of H-Y antigen requires a very complicated immunogenetic assay and is subject to many methodological problems. It is therefore not surprising that Eicher and colleagues have not been able to replicate their results in more recent double-blind procedures (Eicher et al, 1981). Wachtel (personal communication, June 1981), one of the most experienced H-Y antigen researchers, has examined several transsexuals and has not found any H-Y antigen abnormalities. The current consensus, therefore, is that the development of transsexuality cannot be explained by specific deviations in H-Y antigen.

Thus, the diagnosis of transsexualism remains a predominantly psychological task, and the role of the endocrinologist is limited to excluding somatic intersexuality. By contrast, the endocrinologist has a major role in the medical treatment of transsexualism, namely, in those cases that decide to seek sexual reversal by hormone treatment and surgery so that their somatic appearance will be congruent with their desired gender. The medical treatment approach to transsexuality has been justified as a last resort once all forms of psychotherapy are judged as useless or proven unsuccessful in a transsexual patient. The actual hormonal and surgical techniques of sex reversal have been developed out of techniques used for intersex patients. Quite unlike the situation in intersex cases, however, medical treatment of transsexuality is still controversial, mainly because of the lack of a somatic indication of intersexuality which many professionals feel should be a prerequisite to justify such radical medical procedures. The ethical (and theoretical) uneasiness that many professionals feel in relationship to the issue of medical treatment of transsexualism is supported by the lack of a simple set of criteria to predict which patient will benefit from the medical treatment and which will not. Although follow-up studies of well-selected candidates for hormone treatment and surgery have by and large shown remarkably good results (e.g., Money and Ehrhardt, 1970; Hunt and Hampson, 1980; Pauly, 1981; Sørensen, 1981), every major centre has also seen troublesome failures. There are many self-declared transsexuals who either do not fit the diagnostic criteria of transsexualism, or even if they do fit the criteria, can respond to psychotherapy of various sorts and adjust to a different life style, in most cases a homosexual one, that makes medical intervention unnecessary. Where that does not seem possible, secondary psychopathology, especially reactive depression with suicidal risk, are common unless hormone treatment and surgery are performed. Since there is now a black market for sex hormones, many transsexuals (and some male effeminate homosexuals) resort to self-prescription of hormones, sometimes in very large doses. A few have gone so far as to mutilate their own genitalia when they did not find the surgical help wanted. Even such extreme indications of transsexual desire, however, cannot be taken as an indication of the appropriateness of transsexual surgery. Good intentions and the desire to help a desperate individual can, on their own, lead to unwanted consequences, and clinical experience in this area, or at least close collaboration with other experienced professionals, is absolutely necessary.

Most of the key staff of the major university-based centres in the Western world that provide specialized care for patients with gender identity disorder are members of the Harry Benjamin International Gender Dysphoria Association which evolved from a series of international gender dysphoria symposia and was formally founded in 1979. To provide guidance for this particularly difficult area of patient management, the Association developed a set of 'Standards of Care' for the hormonal and surgical sex reassignment of gender dysphoric persons (which in its most recent revision, the draft of March 1981, is being distributed by Dr Paul A. Walker, 1952 Union Street, San Francisco, California 94123, USA). I strongly recommend that any physician involved in the medical management of transsexuals and other gender identity disordered individuals become familiar with the 'Standards' that set *minimal* requirements of care. Concerning endocrine treatment, the 'Standards' require that 'the initiation of hormonal sex reassignment shall be preceded by recommendation for such hormonal therapy made by a clinical behavioral scientist' (c.b.s.) with 'proven competence in general psychotherapy, sex therapy, and gender counseling/therapy'. Further, the 'Standards' reiterate the requirement that the gender disorder has been continuous for at least two years, and that the c.b.s. has knowledge of this, 'independent of the patient's verbal claim', for instance by way of interviews with relatives or friends of the patient. The c.b.s. making these recommendations is required to have known the patient in a psychotherapeutic relationship for at least three months.

In considering hormone administration, the endocrinologist needs to take into consideration the same risk factors or side-effects as in other patients requiring hormone treatment and needs to apprise the patient of those risks. The 'Standards' state that the 'Physician should also make available to the patient (or refer the patient to a facility offering) monitoring relevant blood chemistries and routine physical examinations including, but not limited to, the measurement of SGPT in persons receiving testosterone and the measurement of SGPT, bilirubin, triglycerides, and fasting glucose in persons receiving estrogen'.

Although the issue has not been addressed in the 'Standards', it seems equally important to me that patients who are self-prescribing hormones obtained from the black market are referred to endocrinologists for monitoring of side-effects and risks, medical education, and then, hopefully, supervised endocrine treatment to replace self-prescription. Incidentally, there is also a diagnostic problem here: if there are signs of incongruent pubertal development, especially of gynaecomastia in transsexual males, the endocrinologist needs to take into consideration the possibility of self-prescription of hormones, although the patient may deny this initially. In such patients, particularly careful medical history taking is advised, preferably with involvement of parents, other close relatives, mates or friends.

Hormonal treatment of transsexual patients has a dual goal: to suppress the secondary sex characteristics and functional reminders of the repudiated gender (erection in males, menstruation in females) before gonadectomy, and to further the development of somatic sex characteristics of the desired gender, both before and after gonadectomy, and to ensure their maintenance. A number of papers give specific recommendations for hormonal treatment of transsexual patients (Benjamin, 1966, 1969; Hamburger, 1969; Migeon, 1969, and updated in Money and Walker, 1977; Futterweit, 1980). Systematic studies of hormone treatment effects are rare. Recently, Meyer et al (1981) have compared various forms and dosages of hormonal therapy used in the treatment of non-castrate transsexuals. They found ethinyl oestradiol to be superior to conjugated oestrogen in suppression of testosterone and gonadotrophins but equal in effecting breast growth in males. The changes in physical and hormonal characteristics were the same for 0.1 mg daily and 0.5 mg daily of ethinyl oestradiol. Therefore, they recommended 0.1 mg daily of ethinyl oestradiol for the non-castrate male-to-female transsexual. They found their female-to-male transsexuals well managed with a dose of intramuscular testosterone cypionate of 400 mg per month, usually given as 200 mg every two weeks; the maximal clitoral length reached was usually 4 cm. Higher doses of testosterone did not further increase clitoral length or suppression of gonadotrophin. Consequently, they recommend 200 mg of intramuscular testosterone cypionate every two weeks for the non-castrate female-to-male transsexual. For post-surgical transsexuals, most clinics seem to use maintenance doses of hormones as is customary in other hypogonadal patients. As usual, the minimum dose sufficient to give the clinical effect should be chosen. Note that chronic oestrogen treatment is held responsible for several cancer deaths of male transsexuals, among these two with fatal breast cancer (Symmers, 1968), and ethinyl oestradiol treatment has been suggested as the cause of a pulmonary embolism in a 29-year-old male transsexual (Lehrman, 1976).

SUMMARY

During fetal development of subprimate mammals, sexual differentiation of the genitals and of specific sex-dimorphic brain systems depends on androgens; corresponding sex differences are displayed in prepubertal behaviours as well as in behaviours that depend on activation by pubertal hormones. In human beings, fetal hormones play the same role in genital differentiation. Hormone-dependent structural brain changes are also very likely but have not yet been demonstrated. The corresponding effects of fetal hormones on childhood behaviour have been found both in subhuman primates and in man, while the evidence concerning later behaviour, including sexual orientation, is not yet clear.

The development of gender identity in humans is a cognitive process that has no counterpart in animal behaviour and is unlikely to be based on a specific hormone-sensitive brain system. It appears that the hormone-dependent variations of sex-dimorphic behaviour in childhood can be accommodated within either gender identity, provided that the child's physical appearance is gender adequate and the parental (or other care-givers') rearing style does not interfere with typical gender role development. In intersex individuals, changes in gender identity seem to occur primarily when genital and/or general physical appearance are in conflict with the assigned gender and/or when rearing has been ambiguous. The available descriptions of such changes do not seem compatible with a primarily neuroendocrine explanation. Thus, decisions on sex assignment and reassignment of intersex patients need to be based on expected social and sexual functioning, and the clinical management of such patients must minimize the risk of ambiguous rearing and of the development of a gender-incongruent physical appearance.

The development of a sexual orientation in humans as hetero- or homosexual does not seem to depend on pubertal hormones. The evidence for a role of fetal hormones is suggestive, but the issue is not yet settled. Attempts to implicate the H-Y antigen in the aetiology of transsexuality seem to have failed; psychoendocrine research here parallels that on sexual orientation. Some recent developments in the management of transsexual patients are discussed.

REFERENCES

Abel, G. G. & Blanchard, E. B. (1976) The measurement and generation of sexual arousal. In *Progress in Behavior Modification, Volume II* (Ed.) Hersen, M., Eisler, R. & Miller, P. M. pp. 99-136. New York: Academic Press.

Aono, T., Miyake, A., Kinugasa, T., Kurachi, K & Matsumoto, K. (1978) Absence of positive feedback of oestrogen on LH release in patients with testicular feminization syndrome. *Acta Endocrinologica*, **87**, 259-267.

Bardin, C. W. & Catterall, J. F. (1981) Testosterone: a major determinant of extragenital sexual dimorphism. *Science*, **211**, 1285-1294.

Bell, A. P., Weinberg, M. S. & Hammersmith, S. K. (1981) *Sexual Preference. Its Development in Men and Women*. Bloomington, Indiana: Indiana University Press.

Benjamin, H. (1966) Estrogen therapy. In *The Transsexual Phenomenon*. pp. 92-99. New York: Julian Press.

Benjamin, H. (1969) For the practicing physician: suggestions and guidelines for the management of transsexuals. In *Transsexualism and Sex Reassignment* (Ed.) Green, R. & Money, J. pp. 305-307. Baltimore: Johns Hopkins Press.

Dörner, G. (1967) Tierexperimentelle Untersuchungen zur Frage einer hormonellen Pathogenese der Homosexualität. *Acta Biologica et Medica Germanica,* **19,** 569-584.

Dörner, G. (1968) Hormonal induction and prevention of female homosexuality. *Journal of Endocrinology,* **42,** 163-164.

Dörner, G. (1976) *Hormones and Brain Differentiation.* Amsterdam: Elsevier.

Dörner, G. & Staudt, J. (1972) Vergleichende morphologische Untersuchungen der Hypothalamusdifferenzierung bei Ratte und Mensch. *Endokrinologie,* **59,** 152-155.

Dörner, G., Rohde, W., Seidel, K., Haas, W. & Schott, G. (1976) On the evocability of a positive oestrogen feedback action on LH secretion in transsexual men and women. *Endokrinologie,* **67,** 20-25.

Dörner, G., Geier, Th., Ahrens, L., Krell, L., Münx, G., Sieler, H., Kittner, E. & Müller, H. (1980) Prenatal stress as possible aetiogenetic factor of homosexuality in human males. *Endokrinologie,* **75,** 365-368.

DSM-III *Diagnostic and Statistical Manual of Mental Disorders* (Third Edition) (1980) Washington: American Psychiatric Association.

Ehrhardt, A. A. (1979) Psychosexual adjustment in adolescence in patients with congenital abnormalities of their sex organs. In *Genetic Mechanisms of Sexual Development* (Birth Defects Institute Symposia) (Ed.) Vallet, H. L. & Porter, I. H. pp. 473-484. New York: Academic Press.

Ehrhardt, A. A. & Meyer-Bahlburg, H. F. L. (1981) Effects of prenatal sex hormones on gender-related behavior. *Science,* **211,** 1312-1318.

Ehrhardt, A. A., Evers, K. & Money, J. (1968) Influence of androgen and some aspects of sexually dimorphic behavior in women with the late-treated adrenogenital syndrome. *Johns Hopkins Medical Journal,* **123,** 115-122.

Eicher, W., Spoljar, M., Cleve, H., Murken, J.-D., Richter, K. & Stangel-Rutkowski, S. (1979). H-Y antigen in trans-sexuality. *Lancet,* **ii,** 1137-1138.

Eicher, W., Spoljar, M., Cleve, H., Murken, J.-D., Eiermann, W., Richter, K. & Stengel-Rutkowski, S. (1981) H-Y antigen in transsexuality. Manuscript for presentation at the *Annual Meeting of the International Academy of Sex Research,* Haifa, Israel, June 17-20, 1981.

Ellis, A. (1945) The sexual psychology of human hermaphrodites. *Psychosomatic Medicine,* **7,** 108-125.

Engel, W., Pfäfflin, F. & Wiedeking, C. (1980) H-Y antigen in transsexuality, and how to explain testis differentiation in H-Y antigen-negative males and ovary differentiation in H-Y antigen-positive females. *Human Genetics,* **55,** 315-320.

Forest, M. G., de Peretti, E. & Bertrand, J. (1980) Testicular and adrenal androgens and their binding to plasma proteins in the perinatal period: developmental patterns of plasma testosterone, 4-androstenedione, dehydroepiandrosterone and its sulfate in premature and small for date infants as compared with that of full-term infants. *Journal of Steroid Biochemistry,* **12,** 25-36.

Friedman, R. C., Dyrenfurth, I., Linkie, D., Tendler, R. & Fleiss, J. L. (1977) Hormones and sexual orientation in men. *American Journal of Psychiatry,* **134,** 571-572.

Futterweit, W. (1980) Endocrine management of transsexual. Hormonal profiles of serum prolactin, testosterone, and estradiol. *New York State Journal of Medicine,* **80,** 1260-1264.

Gajdusek, D. C. (1977) Urgent opportunistic observations: the study of changing, transient and disappearing phenomena of medical interest in disrupted primitive human communities. In *Health and Disease in Tribal Societies* (Ed.) Ciba Foundation Symposium 49 (new series). pp. 69-102. Amsterdam: Elsevier Scientific Publishing Company, Excerpta Medica, North-Holland Publishing.

Gartrell, N. K., Loriaux, D. L. & Chase, T. N. (1977) Plasma testosterone in homosexual and heterosexual women. *American Journal of Psychiatry,* **134,** 1117-1119.

Green, R. (1974) *Sexual Identity Conflict in Children and Adults.* New York: Basic Books.

Green, R. (1976) One-hundred ten feminine and masculine boys: behavioral contrasts and demographic similarities. *Archives of Sexual Behavior,* **5,** 425-446.

Green, R. (1979) Childhood cross-gender behavior and subsequent sexual preference. *American Journal of Psychiatry,* **136,** 106-107.

Hamburger, C. (1969) Endocrine treatment of male and female transsexualism. In *Transsexualism and Sex Reassignment* (Ed.) Green, R. & Money, J. pp. 291-304. Baltimore: Johns Hopkins Press.

The Harry Benjamin International Gender Dysphoria Association (1981) *Standards of Care. The Hormonal and Surgical Sex Reassignment of Gender Dysphoric Persons.* Revised Draft (3/81). Unpublished manuscript, distributed by Dr. Paul A. Walker, 1952 Union Street, San Francisco, California 94123, USA.

Haseltine, F. P. & Ohno, S. (1981) Mechanisms of gonadal differentiation. *Science,* **211,** 1272-1277.

Heiman, J. R. (1978) Uses of psychophysiology in the assessment and treatment of sexual dysfunction. In *Handbook of Sex Therapy* (Ed.) LoPiccolo, J. & LoPiccolo, L. pp. 123-135. New York, London: Plenum Press.

Hunt, D. D. & Hampson, J. L. (1980) Follow-up of 17 biologic male transsexuals after sex-reassignment surgery. *American Journal of Psychiatry,* **137,** 432-438.

Imperato-McGinley, J., Guerrero, L., Gautier, T. & Peterson, R. E. (1974) Steroid 5α-reductase deficiency in man: an inherited form of male pseudohermaphroditism. *Science,* **186,** 1213-1215.

Imperato-McGinley, J., Peterson, R. E., Gautier, T. & Sturla, E. (1979) Androgens and the evolution of male-gender identity among male pseudohermaphrodites with 5α-reductase deficiency. *The New England Journal of Medicine,* **300,** 1233-1237.

Karsch, F. J., Dierschke, D. J. & Knobil, E. (1973) Sexual differentiation of pituitary function: apparent difference between primates and rodents. *Science,* **179,** 484-486.

Kinsey, A. C., Pomeroy, W. B. & Martin, C. E. (1948) *Sexual Behavior in the Human Male.* Philadelphia: W. B. Saunders.

Lebovitz, P. S. (1972) Feminine behavior in boys: aspects of its outcome. *American Journal of Psychiatry,* **128,** 1283-1289.

Lehrman, K. L. (1976) Pulmonary embolism in a transsexual man taking diethylstilbestrol. *Journal of the American Medical Association,* **235,** 532-533.

Lewis, M. & Weinraub, M. (1979) Origins of early sex-role development. *Sex Roles,* **5,** 135-153.

MacCulloch, M. J. & Waddington, J. L. (1981) Neuroendocrine mechanisms and the aetiology of male and female homosexuality. *The British Journal of Psychiatry,* **139,** 341-345.

MacLusky, N. J. & Naftolin, F. (1981) Sexual differentiation of the central nervous system. *Science,* **211,** 1294-1303.

McConaghy, N. (1982) Current status of behavior therapy in homosexuality. *Proceedings of the Fifth World Congress of Sexology, Jerusalem, Israel, June 21-26, 1981.* (in press) Amsterdam, Netherlands: Excerpta Medica.

McEwen, B. S. (1981) Neural gonadal steroid actions. *Science,* **211,** 1303-1311.

Meyer, W. J. III, Finkelstein, J. W., Stuart, C. A., Webb, A., Smith, E. R., Payer, A. F. & Walker, P. A. (1981) Physical and hormonal evaluation of transsexual patients during hormonal therapy. *Archives of Sexual Behavior,* **10,** 347-356.

Meyer-Bahlburg, H. F. L. (1977) Sex hormones and male homosexuality in comparative perspective. *Archives of Sexual Behavior,* **6,** 297-325.

Meyer-Bahlburg, H. F. L. (1979) Sex hormones and female homosexuality: a critical examination. *Archives of Sexual Behavior,* **8,** 101-119.

Meyer-Bahlburg, H. F. L. (1980) Hormones and homosexuality. In *Advances in Psychoneuroendocrinology. The Psychiatric Clinics of North America,* **3** (2), 349-364. Philadelphia: W. B. Saunders.

Migeon, C. J. (1969) Appendix: therapy for the control of postcastration symptoms. In *Transsexualism and Sex Reassignment* (Ed.) Green, R. & Money, J. pp. 353-354. Baltimore: Johns Hopkins Press.

Migeon, C. J., Rivarola, M. A. & Forest, M. G. (1969) Studies of androgens in male transsexual subjects; effects of estrogen therapy. In *Transsexualism and Sex Reassignment* (Ed.) Green, R. & Money, J. pp. 203-211. Baltimore: Johns Hopkins Press.

Money, J. (1968) *Sex Errors of the Body.* Baltimore: Johns Hopkins Press.

Money, J. (1969) Sex reassignment as related to hermaphroditism and transsexualism. In *Transsexualism and Sex Reassignment* (Ed.) Green, R. & Money, J. pp. 91-113. Baltimore: Johns Hopkins Press.

Money, J. (1975) Psychologic counseling: hermaphroditism. In *Endocrine and Genetic Diseases of Childhood and Adolescence* (Ed.) Gardner, L. I. pp. 609-618. Philadelphia: W. B. Saunders.

Money, J. & Ehrhardt, A. A. (1970) Transsexuelle nach Geschlechtswechsel: Partnerbeziehung, Beruf, Straffälligkeit, psychiatrische Behandlung und subjektive Bewertung des Geschlechtswechsels. *Beiträge zur Sexualforschung,* **49,** 70-87.

Money, J. & Ehrhardt, A. A. (1972) *Man & Woman, Boy & Girl.* Baltimore, London: Johns Hopkins University Press.

Money, J. & Russo, A. J. (1979) Homosexual outcome of discordant gender identity/role in childhood: longitudinal follow-up. *Journal of Pediatric Psychology,* **4,** 29-41.

Money, J. & Walker, P. A. (1977) Counseling the transsexual. In *Handbook of Sexology* (Ed.) Money, J. & Musaph, H. pp. 1289-1301. Amsterdam, London, New York: Elsevier/North Holland Biomedical Press.

Money, J., Hampson, J. G. & Hampson, J. L. (1955a) Hermaphroditism: recommendations concerning assignment of sex, change of sex, and psychologic management. *Bulletin of the Johns Hopkins Hospital,* **97,** 284-300.

Money, J., Hampson, J. G. & Hampson, J. L. (1955b) An examination of some basic sexual concepts: the evidence of human hermaphroditism. *Bulletin of The Johns Hopkins Hospital,* **97,** 301-319.

Money, J., Hampson, J. G. & Hampson, J. L. (1956) Sexual incongruities and psychopathology: the evidence of human hermaphroditism. *Bulletin of The Johns Hopkins Hospital,* **98,** 43-57.

Müller, D., Orthner, H., Roeder, F., König, A., Bosse, K. & Kloos, G. (1974) Einfluss von Hypothalamusläsionen auf Sexualverhalten und gonadotrope Funktion beim Menschen. Bericht über 23 Fälle. In *Endocrinology of Sex: Differentiation and Neuroendocrine Regulation in the Hypothalamo-Hypophyseal-Gonadal System* (Ed.) Dörner, G. pp. 80-105. Leipzig: Johann Ambrosius Barth.

Naftolin, F. & Butz, E. (Ed.) (1981) Sexual dimorphism. *Science,* **211** (4488), 1261-1324.

Pauly, I. B. (1981) Outcome of sex reassignment surgery for transsexuals. *Australian and New Zealand Journal of Psychiatry,* **15,** 45-51.

Peterson, R. E., Imperato-McGinley, J., Gautier, T. & Sturla, E. (1977) Male pseudohermaphroditism due to steroid 5α-reductase deficiency. *The American Journal of Medicine,* **62,** 170-191.

Pfaff, D. W. (1980) *Estrogens and Brain Function. Neural Analysis of a Hormone-Controlled Mammalian Reproductive Behavior.* New York, Heidelberg, Berlin: Springer-Verlag.

Rekers, G. A., Crandall, B. F., Rosen, A. C. & Bentler, P. M. (1979) Genetic and physical studies of male children with psychological gender disturbances. *Psychological Medicine,* **9,** 373-375.

Rubin, R. T., Reinisch, J. M. & Haskett, R. F. (1981) Postnatal gonadal steroid effects on human behavior. *Science,* **211,** 1318-1324.

Saghir, M. T. & Robins, E. R. (1973) *Male and Female Homosexuality: A Comprehensive Investigation.* Baltimore: Williams and Wilkins.

Schmidt, G. & Schorsch, E. (1981) Psychosurgery of sexually deviant patients: review and analysis of new empirical findings. *Archives of Sexual Behaviour,* **10,** 301-323.

Seyler, L. E., Canalis, E., Spare, S. & Reichlin, S. (1978) Abnormal gonadotropin secretory responses to LRH in transsexual women after diethylstilbestrol priming. *Journal of Clinical Endocrinology and Metabolism,* **47,** 176-183.

Sórensen, T. (1981) A follow-up study of operated transsexual females. *Acta Psychiatrica Scandinavica,* **64,** 50-64.

Spoljar, M., Eicher, W., Eiermann, W. & Cleve, H. (1981) H-Y antigen expression in different tissues from transsexuals. *Human Genetics,* **57,** 52-57.

Steiner, R. A., Clifton, D. K., Spies, H. G. & Resko, J. A. (1976) Sexual differentiation and feedback control of luteinizing hormone secretion in the rhesus monkey. *Biology of Reproduction,* **15,** 206-212.

Symmers, W. S. (1968) Carcinoma of breast in transsexual individuals after surgical and hormonal interference with the primary and secondary sex characteristics. *British Medical Journal,* **ii,** 83-85.

Toran-Allerand, C. D. (1980) Sex steroids and the development of the newborn mouse hypothalamus and preoptic area in vitro: II. Morphological correlates and hormonal specificity. *Brain Research,* **189,** 413-427.

Van Look, P. F. A., Hunter, W. M., Corker, C. S. & Baird, D. T. (1977) Failure of positive feedback in normal men and subjects with testicular feminization. *Clinical Endocrinology,* ₒ **7,** 353-366.

Wålinder, J. & Thuwe, I. (1975) *A Social-Psychiatric Follow-up Study of 24 Sex-Reassigned Transsexuals.* Göteborg, Sweden: Scandinavian University Books; Akademiförlaget.

Ward, I. L. (1972) Prenatal stress feminizes and demasculinizes the behavior of males. *Science,* **175,** 82-84.

Ward, I. L. (1977) Exogenous androgen activates female behavior in noncopulating, prenatally stressed male rats. *Journal of Comparative and Physiological Psychology,* **91,** 465-471.

Wilson, G. D. & Fulford, K. W. M. (1977) Sexual behaviour, personality and hormonal characteristics of heterosexual, homosexual and bisexual men. In *Love and Attraction* (Ed.) Cook, M. & Wilson, G. pp. 387-394. Oxford: Pergamon Press.

Wilson, J. D., George, F. W. & Griffin, J. E. (1981) The hormonal control of sexual development. *Science,* **211,** 1278-1284.

Wolf, T. P. (1968) *Geschlechtswechsel bei Hermaphroditen.* Unpublished inaugural dissertation, Ruprecht-Karl Universität, Heidelberg, FR Germany.

Zuger, B. (1978) Effeminate behavior present in boys from childhood: ten additional years of follow-up. *Comprehensive Psychiatry,* **19,** 363-369.

6

The Sexual Development of Boys with the Chromosome Constitution 47,XXY (Klinefelter's Syndrome)

SHIRLEY G. RATCLIFFE

INTRODUCTION

The clinical recognition of Klinefelter's syndrome at birth or in childhood remains unusual, and hence information concerning the early stages of its natural history has not been generally available (Williams, 1981). However, the establishment of the newborn chromosome surveys in the 1960s led to the identification of over 100 newborn male infants with a non-mosaic sex chromosome constitution, 47,XXY. These surveys were carried out in North America (Sergovich et al, 1969; Lubs and Ruddle, 1970; Bell and Corey, 1974; Hamerton et al, 1975; Goad, Robinson and Puck, 1976; Walzer and Gerald, 1977), in Britain (Jacobs et al, 1974; Buckton et al, 1980) and in Denmark (Nielsen and Sillesen, 1975). Approximately 90 of these boys have received detailed study from birth, and in this chapter an attempt will be made to collate the information from these several studies with other data from the literature in order to draw a picture of the early development of these boys. Most of the information relates to physical rather than psychosexual development as it is only comparatively recently that techniques of interview have been developed enabling this area to be scrutinized and, not surprisingly, few studies have been carried out in childhood or adolescence.

CLINICAL FINDINGS AT BIRTH

Body size. Careful measurement showed that the XXY infant is smaller at birth than male controls, but is almost identical to female controls in respect of birth weight, birth length and head circumference (Ratcliffe, Axworthy and Ginsborg, 1979).

The genitalia. The majority of XXY infants identified by newborn screening have had no abnormality of the penis, but Nielsen and Sillesen (1975) described one infant with 'rather a small penis' and one with hypospadias. However, incomplete descent of one or both testes occurred in 6.3

per cent compared with an incidence of 0.87 per cent in 4480 carefully-examined infants (Leonard et al, 1979). In all infants the testes were normal in size and consistency. Inguinal herniae were unusually frequent, being present in four of 63 infants.

GROWTH OF THE GENITALIA DURING CHILDHOOD

Laron and Hochman (1971) noted that eight of nine children with Klinefelter's syndrome seen in an endocrine clinic had small testes, despite statements in several textbooks that the clinical signs of the condition were undetectable before puberty. His cases ranged from two to twelve years of age, the testicular volumes varied from 0.5 to 1.5 ml and were smaller than normal values established for Israeli children by Zilka and Laron (1969). The 1981 edition of Williams' 'Textbook of Endocrinology' states that small testes may be noticeable from the age of three years.

In the Edinburgh study of 20 boys with the sex chromosome constitution 47,XXY testicular volume has been measured serially since birth using Prader's orchidometer (Prader, 1966). Fourteen of the 20 boys were considered to have reduced size of the testes, some being only 0.5 ml in volume and soft in consistency from the age of six months. Mean values for the group are given in Table 1; these values show a gradual increase throughout childhood, accelerating between the ages of 10.5 and 11.0 years. Figure 1 shows a comparison in the growth of the testes in a pair of twins, one of whom had an XXY karyotype. To date only three boys have shown signs of the commencement of puberty, and this occurred at ages 11.0, 11.5 and 12.5 years.

Table 1. *Testicular volume by age in 47,XXY boys*

	Age in years										
	0.25	0.5	1.0	2.0	3.0	5.0	7.0	8.0	10.0	11.0	12.0
Mean volume (mls)	0.41	0.42	0.45	0.55	0.65	0.66	1.10	1.01	1.32	2.25	3.30
n	9	12	14	13	13	8	6	4	7	6	4

The Toronto group noted small size of the testes in only three of the 28 boys studied longitudinally (Stewart et al, 1979). However, the orchidometer they used was a copy of Prader's original instrument and gave readings somewhat in excess of true size. On the other hand Robinson et al (1979) in Denver found testicular size to be below Prader's mean values for age in 15 of 16 boys with the XXY karyotype.

As regards the size of the penis, most studies record only a minority of boys to have a penis smaller than average. Robinson et al (1979) reported that only three of their 16 cases had values for stretched penile length below the norms of Zilka and Laron (1969). In the Edinburgh group six boys out of 20 had reduced size of the penis.

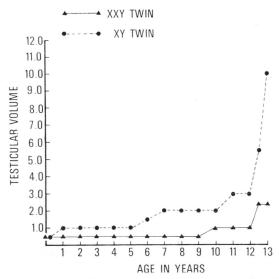

Figure 1. Comparison of testicular growth in a pair of twins, one XXY.

The successful use of locally-applied 2 per cent testosterone cream was described by Immergut et al (1971) and Jacobs, Kaplan and Gitts (1975) for microphallus in boys prior to surgery for hypospadias and was shown experimentally (Jacobs, Judd and Gitts, 1977) to produce increased weight of the whole penis in rats. This treatment was used in the Edinburgh cases with the necessary precaution that only the prescribed amount, containing approximately 3 mg of testosterone, was applied to the shaft and glans of the penis nightly. This resulted in rapid growth of the penis over three to four months until normal size was reached in all cases, but we have no experience as to its efficacy over the age of eight years.

PUBERTY

As yet there is insufficient information from the newborn studies to comment on the age of onset of puberty. The Zurich study of cases of Klinefelter's syndrome referred to an endocrine clinic (Schibler et al, 1974) found that the age of onset of puberty was slightly later than that of Zurich males, but the difference was not significant at the 5 per cent level.

Ratcliffe et al (1982) examined 12 boys with an XXY karyotype between the ages of 16 and 18 years. These boys had been identified in the newborn sex chromatin survey of MacLean et al (1964), and controls who were matched for age, social class, and birth order were selected from the same newborn population. Comparison of sexual development in the two groups showed that although pubic hair growth and genital development were somewhat less advanced in the XXY boys, they were not significantly so. However, the difference in the size of the testes between the XXY boys and the controls was highly significant, most of the cases having testes of 3 to 5 ml volume while the controls had testicular volumes of 12 to 15 ml. It was noted, however, that one boy with an XXY karyotype had testes of 12 ml volume bilaterally and of normal consistency, so that his testes were indistinguishable from those of the controls on palpation. However, he had raised serum levels of gonadotrophins, indicating that some degree of testicular dysfunction was present. It would seem likely in this case that tubular development was considerably better than average in an XXY male, and that caution is required in relation to the prognosis for sterility usually given to patients with Klinefelter's syndrome.

BODY PROPORTIONS

In XXY boys an increase in leg length is present by three years of age in many cases (Ratcliffe et al, 1982) and increased fat deposition on the hips may be apparent by the age of ten years (Figures 2 and 3). However, in many boys the body proportions are undisturbed (Figure 4).

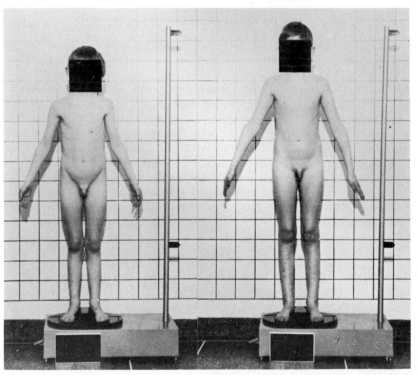

Figure 2. Eight-year-old twins, the taller of whom has an XXY sex chromosome constitution. Increased leg length and smaller scrotal size is noticeable.

PSYCHOSEXUAL DEVELOPMENT

Personality tests and assessment of psychosexual development were also carried out in the adolescent group of boys in Edinburgh (Bancroft, Axworthy and Ratcliffe, 1982). On the Cattell High School Personality

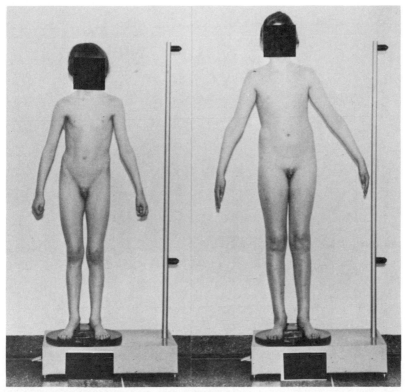

Figure 3. The same pair of twins as in Figure 2, now aged 10 years. In the XXY twin the penis is proportionally smaller, there is increased fat deposition on the hips and a more marked increase in leg length.

Questionnaire the boys rated themselves as more tender-minded, appre-hensive and insecure, and they achieved lower scores on the subscale 'mental capacity and ability to abstract'. They reported less sexual interest in girls and a later onset of masturbation (14.3 compared with 13.4 years in the controls); however, the number who did masturbate and the frequency of masturbation was not different between the two groups.

On the Bem sex role inventory the XXY boys obtained lower scores for masculinity than the controls, but their scores for femininity and social desirability were also lower, although to a lesser extent. This combination would seem to indicate a general lowering of self-esteem. There was no evidence of increased homosexuality.

HORMONE STUDIES

Prenatal. With the increasing use of amniocentesis, fetuses with the XXY karyotype are being recognized in the second trimester of pregnancy. Mean et al (1981) measured testosterone levels in amniotic fluid, using

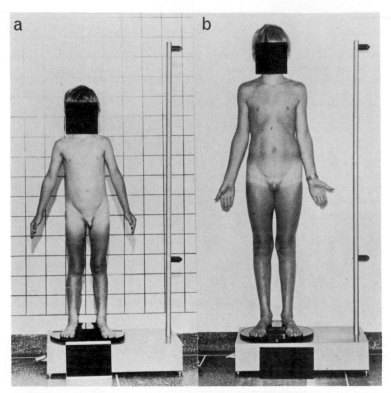

Figure 4. Two boys, aged (a) five and (b) eight years, with XXY sex chromosome constitutions and with normal body proportions. The older boy has scars of bilateral orchidoplexies for undescended testes.

radioimmunoassay in one XXY fetus at 16 weeks, and found a level of 277 pg/ml. The range found in 29 chromosomally normal male fetuses was 155 to 730 pg/ml, mean 327 ± 25 SEM pg/ml. They concluded that in this single case there was no evidence of deficiency of testosterone production.

At birth. Sørensen et al (1981) measured cord blood testosterone by radio-immunoassay in two 47,XXY infants and reported levels of 1.0 and 1.4 nmol/l, which were lower than those found in two control infants at 1.7 and 2.1 nmol/l. In a third infant with mosaicism 46,XY/47,XXY they obtained a level of 1.3 nmol/l (control 1.7 nmol/l). On the basis of results of paired significance tests they concluded that testicular function was reduced during the last part of fetal life in Klinefelter's syndrome, as it was in adult life. However, using the same technique Forest, Cathiard and Bertrand (1973) had reported a mean cord blood level of testosterone of 1.17 (SD 0.33) nmol/l (33.8 ± 9.5 ng per 10 ml) from 35 normal male infants, while Ratcliffe and Corker found a mean value of 1.32 (SD 0.75) nmol/l in the cord blood of ten normal male infants. By comparison with these figures the levels in Sørensen's cases would not be remarkable.

Neonatal. Following the finding by Forest, Cathiard and Bertrand (1973) of a dramatic rise in serum testosterone in normal male infants between three and six weeks of life, Ratcliffe (1976) reported the findings in six XXY infants; these are shown in Table 2. The levels found were not significantly different from controls, or from the levels found in normal infants by Forest and Cathiard. On these results it was not considered justifiable to treat such infants with testosterone at this age.

Table 2. *Serum testosterone in 47,XXY infants and controls (nmols/l) (numbers of infants tested in brackets)*

Age (days)	47,XXY	Controls R[a]	Controls F[b]
5-7	1.63 ± 0.59	1.60 ± 0.42	1.13 ± 0.46
	(5)	(4)	(8)
27-45	7.69 ± 1.24	7.28 ± 2.39	7.42 ± 2.18
	(6)	(19)	(6)

[a]Ratcliffe and Corker, personal communication
[b]Forest and Cathiard (1975)

Prepubertal. Illig et al (1975) described the result of synthetic LH-RH stimulation in seven prepubertal boys with Klinefelter's syndrome. In six boys both basal and peak values for LH and FSH were normal, the remaining boy had gonadotrophin levels in the pubertal range at the age of eleven years and responded actively to stimulation. de Behar et al (1975) also reported normal levels of LH and FSH in eight prepubertal boys with Klinefelter's syndrome and noted that following LH-RH stimulation the FSH increased by 221 per cent, LH by 261 per cent. However, in pubertal subjects the FSH response was reduced, being only 13 per cent greater than the base level.

Of the 43 infants with the karyotype 47,XXY identified in the Toronto study of Bell and Corey (1974), 28 were seen for follow-up by Stewart et al (1979), who reported that 'testosterone levels were below 20 μg/dl (0.654 nmol/l) in all subjects tested', but gave no indication of the numbers of tests carried out or the precise values obtained. Robinson et al (1979) give results in two prepubertal boys who had basal testosterone levels of 10 and 12 ng/dl (0.347 and 0.416 nmol/l), rising after HCG stimulation to 54 and 85 ng/dl (1.87 and 2.95 nmol/l) respectively, which was considered a normal prepubertal response. Furthermore the response to LH-RH stimulation was also within the normal range. Salbenblatt et al (1981) reported random serum testosterone levels from four XXY boys age 11 to 13 from Robinson's study which were also within the normal values of Winter (1978), as they were in three additional referred cases. Results from the Edinburgh cases are shown in Figure 5 and show that elevation of gonadotrophins appear around age 11 years.

Puberty. Ratcliffe et al (1982) investigated twelve 47,XXY boys who had been identified in the newborn sex chromatin survey of Maclean et al (1964)

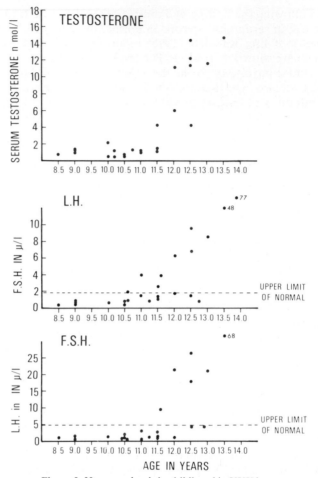

Figure 5. Hormone levels in childhood in XXY boys.

and compared the findings with those from twelve chromosomally normal boys from the same newborn population when they were between the ages of 16 and 18 years. Testosterone levels were significantly lower at 14.06 (SD 5.17) nmol/l compared with the mean level in the controls of 21.60 (SD 7.74) nmol/l. LH was moderately elevated at 19.64 (SD 13.10) U/l compared with the control mean level of 5.28 (SD 2.56) U/l, while elevation of FSH was highly significant ($P < 0.002$), the 47,XXY boys having a mean level of 37.56 (SD 22.40) U/l compared with 4.57 (SD 4.11) U/l in the control boys. The findings from birth to age 18 are summarized in Figure 6.

TESTICULAR PATHOLOGY

Owing to the difficulty of obtaining normative data ·the full range of development of the postnatal human testis has not yet been well established.

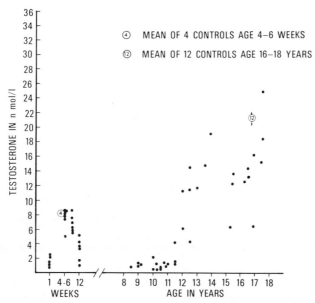

Figure 6. Serum testosterone in XXY boys aged one week to 18 years.

The useful review of their personal experience by Charny, Conston and Meranze (1952) is based on small numbers, especially in the younger age groups. The basis of a quantitative assessment was laid down by Mancini, Narbaitz and Laviem (1960) but is not in widespread use as yet; most reports of testicular histology in Klinefelter's syndrome are mainly descriptive. Murken et al (1974) reported the histological findings in a fetus with the karyotype 47,XXY, aborted at 20 weeks gestation, in whom the testes were found in the inguinal canal. They noted pronounced hyperplasia of the Leydig cells, hypoplastic and hypotrophic tubules, and highly reduced germinal epithelium. By contrast much less marked changes were found in the biopsy of the right testis of a four-week-old infant with the karyotype 47,XXY from the Edinburgh study, illustrated in Figure 7. The baby underwent surgery for an inguinal hernia and a testicular biopsy was obtained at the time. Numerous germ cells and immature Sertoli cells are present, and the Leydig cells appear normal. However, quantitative assay of spermatogonia indicated that they were less numerous than expected compared with Mancini's controls.

Mikamo et al (1968) have made the most useful contribution to our knowledge of the histology of the testes in this condition by describing testicular biopsies from three infants, age three, four and twelve months, who were identified by sex chromatin screening at birth. In the three-month-old infant quantitative study revealed that the number of spermatogonia in each tubule was reduced, being only 21 per cent of the control value of Mancini, Narbaitz and Lavieri (1960). However, tubular diameter and undifferentiated Sertoli cells were unaffected. The four-month-old infant had a small penis and incomplete descent of the right testis. Biopsy of

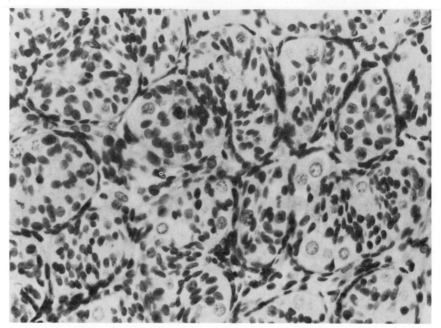

Figure 7. Testicular biopsy in a four-week-old infant with an XXY sex chromosome constitution. (Haematoxylin and eosin, × 380.)

the left testis showed a greater reduction of spermatogonia than in the three-month-old case. By twelve months of age the biopsy of the third case showed only 0.1 per cent of the expected number of spermatogonia.

These findings, taken in conjunction with the more normal appearance at four weeks of age, are suggestive of an active progression of changes during the first year of life. Mikamo et al (1968) make the interesting comment that similar histological changes are found in chromatin negative and chromatin positive forms of Klinefelter's syndrome in adult life, so it is difficult to postulate that they are initiated by the presence of an additional X chromosome in the cells of the testis.

Lawrence and Yuceoglu (1961) reported only minimal irregularity of tubular diameter in a testicular biopsy from a ten-month-old child with normal genitalia and a 47,XXY karyotype, but no quantitative studies were undertaken.

A double pathology was present in the case of Lanman et al (1960) with Down's Syndrome in addition to an XXY sex chromosome complement, making absence of the germinal epithelium difficult to evaluate. However, the small number of Leydig cells and the absence of lumen in the tubules would not be unusual in a ten-month-old infant. Figure 8 shows the biopsy from an eight-year-old XXY boy at the time of surgery for undescended testes, when the histological findings (Dr Neil MacLean) were described as indistinguishable from those of undescended testis alone.

Ferguson-Smith et al (1959) have described the testicular histology in mid childhood in eight mentally defective chromatin positive boys aged seven to

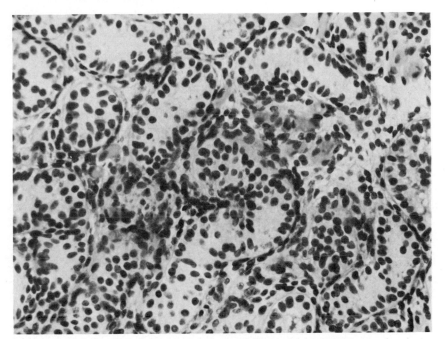

Figure 8. Testicular biopsy in an eight-year-old boy with an XXY sex chromosome constitution. (Haematoxylin and eosin, × 380.)

twelve years. It was noted that their testes seemed smaller than normal, and all showed abnormal testicular histology, the main features being smaller seminiferous tubules and a reduction, amounting to absence in some cases, of spermatogonia. There were some normal tubules but these never made up more than 20 per cent of the total number. The lesions appeared to advance with age so that in the twelve-year-old boy there was virtually complete absence of germinal cells and commencing tubular hyalinization. These authors also noted that a similar deficiency of germ cells is also seen in true crypto-orchidism, making evaluation of the changes difficult when the two conditions are combined. Somewhat more advanced changes approaching the adult pattern were seen in the fifteen-year-old (but prepubertal) boy described by Barr et al (1959), where the tissue consisted mainly of hyalinized tubular remnants, devoid of epithelium, surrounded by loose, poorly organized connective tissue. There were occasional groups of seminiferous tubules which were smaller than normal, with moderate thickening of the tunica propria. This case is probably an example of the 48,XXXY type as two Barr bodies were present in 54 per cent of the cells.

CONCLUSIONS

The use of newborn screening in the identification of XXY boys has enabled the natural history to be described in more detail than previously, but still requires supplementation by more extensive data collected with rigorous comparison to adequate controls. Careful clinical examination reveals differences in the size and consistency of the testes in a proportion of young XXY boys, but hormone assays have not proved helpful, due possibly to their lack of sensitivity in the range of testosterone levels found in early childhood. The development of greater sensitivity in the assays is essential if the contribution of sex hormone deficiency to the physical and behavioural alterations is to be clarified.

Walzer et al (1978) found that XXY boys under the age of three years 'showed lower activity levels, were more mild in the energy content of their responsiveness, responded to novel stimuli by withdrawal, (and) were more pliant in their social interactions'. The possibility that these characteristics were related to lower testosterone levels was not explored but would be important for the future development of these boys. Ideally blood blot assays during the first three years of life, followed by timed urine assays throughout early childhood, would enable sex hormone deficiency to be detected and, if found, treated.

The delayed speech development and small but significant cognitive deficit are clearly due to other than hormonal mechanisms. These problems can be ameliorated by speech therapy and appropriate educational help, leaving the major area for research in the life of XXY boy in the lap of the endocrinologist.

REFERENCES

Bancroft, J., Axworthy, D. & Ratcliffe, S. G. (1982) The personality and psycho-sexual development of boys with 47,XXY chromosome constitution. *Journal of Child Psychology and Psychiatry,* **23,** 169-180.
Barr, M. L., Shaver, E. L., Carr, D. H. & Plunker, E. R. (1959) An unusual sex chromatin pattern in three mentally deficient subjects. *Journal of Mental Deficiency Research,* **3,** 78-87.
Bell, A. G. & Corey, P. N. (1974) A sex chromatin and Y body survey of Toronto newborns. *Canadian Journal of Genetics and Cytology,* **16,** 239-250.
Buckton, K. E., O'Riordan, M., Ratcliffe, S. G., Slight, J., Mitchell, M., McBeath, S., Keay, A., Barr, D. & Short, M. (1980) A G band study of chromosome in liveborn infants. *Annals of Human Genetics, London,* **43,** 227-239.
Charny, C. W., Conston, A. S. & Meranze, D. R. (1952) Development of the testes. *Fertility and Sterility,* **3,** 461-479.
de Behar, B. R., Mendilaharzu, H., Rivarola, M. A. & Bergada, C. (1975) Gonadotropin secretion in prepubertal and pubertal primary hypogonadism: response to LH RH. *Journal of Clinical Endocrinology and Metabolism,* **41,** 1070-1075.
Ferguson-Smith, M. A. (1959) The prepubertal testicular lesion in chromatin positive Klinefelter's syndrome (primary micro-orchidism) as seen in mentally handicapped children. *Lancet,* **i,** 219-222.
Forest, M. G. & Cathiard, A. M. (1975) Pattern of plasma testosterone and Δ^4-androstenedione in normal newborns: evidence for testicular activity at birth. *Journal of Clinical Endocrinology and Metabolism,* **41,** 977-980.
Forest, M. G., Cathiard, A. M. & Bertrand, J. A. (1973) Evidence of testicular activity in early infancy. *Journal of Clinical Endocrinology and Metabolism,* **37,** 148-151.
Goad, W. D., Robinson, A. & Puck, T. T. (1976) The incidence of aneuploidy in a human population. *American Journal of Human Genetics,* **28,** 62-68.
Hamerton, J. L., Canning, N., Ray, M. & Smith, S. (1975) A cytogenetic survey of 14,069 newborn infants. I. Incidence of chromosome abnormalities. *Clinical Genetics,* **8,** 223-243.

Illig, R., Tolksdorf, M., Mürset, G. & Prader, A. (1975) LH and FSH response to synthetic LH-RH in children and adolescents with Turner's and Klinefelter's syndrome. *Helvetia Paediatrica Acta,* **30,** 221-231.

Immergut, M., Boldus, R., Yannone, E., Bunce, R. & Flocks, R. (1971) The local application of testosterone cream to the prepubertal phallus. *Journal of Urology,* **105,** 905-906.

Jacobs, P. A., Melville, M., Ratcliffe, S. G.; Keay, A. J. & Syme, J. (1974) A cytogenetic survey of 11,680 newborn infants. *Annals of Human Genetics,* **37,** 359-376.

Jacobs, S. C., Kaplan, G. W. & Gittes, R. F. (1975) Topical testosterone therapy for penile growth. *Urology,* **6,** 708-710.

Jacobs, S. C., Judd, H. M. & Gittes, R. F. (1977) Penile growth: topical versus systemic testosterone therapy in rats. *Journal of Endocrinology,* **73,** 189-190.

Lanman, J. T., Sklarin, B. S., Cooper, H. L. & Hirschhorn, K. (1960) Klinefelter's syndrome in a 10-month-old Mongolian Idiot. *New England Journal of Medicine,* **263,** 881-890.

Laron, Z. & Hochman, I. H. (1971) Small testes in prepubertal boys with Klinefelter's syndrome. *Journal of Clinical Endocrinology,* **32,** 671-672.

Lawrence, R. & Yuceoglu, A. M. (1961) Seminiferous tubule dysgenesis: a case of Klinefelter's syndrome in a ten-month-old child. *American Journal of Diseases of Children,* **101,** 635-638.

Leonard, M. F., Schowalter, J. E., Landy, G., Ruddle, F. H. & Lubs, H. A. (1979) Chromosomal abnormalities in the New Haven newborn study: a prospective study of development of children with sex chromosome abnormalities. In *Sex Chromosome Aneuploidy: Prospective Studies in Children* (Ed.) Robinson, A., Lubs, H. A. & Bergsma, D. *Birth Defects Original Article Series,* **xv,** pp. 115-159. New York: Alan R. Liss.

Lubs, H. A. & Ruddle, F. H. (1970) Applications of quantitative karyotypy to chromosome variations in 4,400 consecutive newborns. In *Human Population Cytogenetics* (Ed.) Jacobs, P., Price, W. H. & Law, P. pp. 120-142. Edinburgh: University Press.

MacLean, N., Harnden, D. G., Court Brown, W. M., Bond, J. & Mantle, D. J. (1964) Sex chromosome abnormalities in newborn babies. *Lancet,* **i,** 286-290.

Mancini, R. E., Narbaitz, R. & Lavieri, J. C. (1960) The origin and development of the germinative epithelium and Sertoli cells in the human testis: cytological, cytochemical and quantitative study. *Anatomical Record,* **136,** 477-483.

Mean, F., Pescia, G., Vajda, D., Felber, J. P. & Magrini (1981) Amniotic fluid testosterone in pre-natal sex determination. *Journal de Genetique Humaine,* **29** (4), 441-447.

Mikamo, K., Aguercif, M., Hazechi, P. & Martin du Pan, R. (1968) Chromatin positive Klinefelter's syndrome. *Fertility and Sterility,* **19,** 731-739.

Murken, J-D., Stengel-Rutkowski, S., Walther, J-U., Westenfelder, S. R., Remberger, K. H. & Zimmer, F. (1974) Klinefelter's syndrome in a fetus. *Lancet,* **ii,** 171.

Nielsen, J., & Sillesen, I. (1975) The incidence of chromosome aberrations among 11,148 newborn children. *Humangenetik,* **30,** 1-12.

Prader, A. (1966) Testicular size: assessment and clinical importance. *Triangle,* **7,** 240-243.

Ratcliffe, S. G. (1976) The development of children with sex chromosome abnormalities. *Proceedings of the Royal Society of Medicine,* **69,** 189-191.

Ratcliffe, S. G., Axworthy, D. & Ginsborg, A. (1979) The Edinburgh study of growth and development of children with sex chromosome abnormalities. In *Sex Chromosome Aneuploidy: Prospective Studies in Children* (Ed.) Robinson, A., Lubs, H. A. & Bergsma, D. Birth Defects Original Article Series, **XV** (1), 243-260. New York: Alan R. Liss.

Ratcliffe, S. G., Bancroft, J., Axworthy, D. & McLaren, W. (1982a) Klinefelter's syndrome in adolescence. *Archives of Disease in Childhood,* **57,** 6-12.

Ratcliffe, S. G., Tierney, I., Nshaho, J., Smith, L., Springbett, A. & Callan, S. (1982b) Sex Chromosome Aneuploidy: prospective studies in children No. 2 (in press).

Robinson, A., Puck, M., Pennington, B., Borelli, J. & Hudson, M. (1979) Abnormalities of the sex chromosomes: a prospective study on randomly identified newborns. In *Sex Chromosome Aneuploidy: prospective studies in children.* (Ed.) Robinson, A., Lubs, H. A. & Bergsma, D. Birth Defects Original Article Series Volume **XV,** No. 1. pp. 203-241. New York: Alan R. Liss.

Salbenblatt, J. A., Bender, B. G., Puck, M. H., Robinson, A. & Webber, M. L. (1981) Development of eight pubertal males with 47 XXY karyotype. *Clinical Genetics,* **20,** 141-146.

Schibler, D., Brook, C. G. D., Kind, H. P., Zachmann, M. & Prader, (1974) Growth and body proportions in 54 boys and men with Klinefelter's syndrome. *Helvetica Paediatrica Acta,* **29,** 325-333.

Sergovich, F., Valentine, G. H., Chen, A. T. L., Kinch, R. A. H. & Smout, M. S. (1969) Chromosome aberrations in 2159 consecutive newborn babies. *New England Journal of Medicine,* **280,** 851-855.

Sørensen, K., Nielsen, J., Wohlert, M., Bennett, P. & Johnsen, S. G. (1981) Serum testosterone of boys with karyotype 47,XXY (Klinefelter's syndrome) at birth. *Lancet,* **i,** 1112-1113.

Stewart, D. A., Netley, C. T., Bailey, J. D., Haka-Ikse, K., Platt, J., Holland, W. & Cripps, M. (1979) Growth and development of children with X and Y chromosome aneuploidy: a prospective study. In *Sex Chromosome Aneuploidy. Prospective Studies in Children* (Ed.) Robinson, A., Lubs, H. & Bergsma, D. pp. 75-114. Birth Defects Original Article series Vol. XV, No. 1. New York: Alan R. Liss.

Walzer, S. & Gerald, P. S. (1977) A chromosome survey of 13,751 male newborns. In *Population Cytogenetics* (Ed.) Hook, E. B. & Porter, I. H. pp. 45-61. New York: Academic Press.

Walzer, S., Wolff, P. H., Bowen, D., Silbert, A., Bashir, A. S., Gerald, P. S. & Richmond, J. B. (1978) A method for the longitudinal study of behavioral development in infants and children: the early development of XXY children. *Journal of Child Psychology & Psychiatry,* **19,** 213-229.

Williams, R. H. (Ed) (1981) *Textbook of Endocrinology,* 6th edition. Philadelphia: W. B. Saunders.

Winter, J. D. S. (1978) Prepubertal and pubertal endocrinology. In *Human Growth* (Ed.) Faulkner, F. & Tanner, J. M., Vol. **2.** New York: Plenum Publishing.

Zilka, E. & Laron, Z. (1969) Norm determination for testicular size in childhood and adolescence in Israel. *Harefuah,* **77,** 511-513.

7

Vascular Mechanisms Involved in Erection and Erectile Disorders

GORM WAGNER

INTRODUCTION

The vascular mechanisms involved in the penile erection are not fully understood. The process consists of four phases — flaccidity, tumescence, erection, and detumescence — and depends on precise neural control of the highly specialized vascular organs, the two corpora cavernosa and the spongiose body. The latter contains the urethra and, in the form of the glans, covers the distal end of the cavernous bodies (Wagner and Green, 1981).

The main theories to account for these four phases will be dealt with in this chapter, together with such pathological conditions that may be caused by defects in the vascular function.

THE MECHANISM OF ERECTION

As yet our knowledge concerning the neural regulation of these vascular mechanisms is meagre. The peripheral, motor nerves are recognized and well described, but we are largely ignorant of the interneuronal transmission system, and the function of neuropeptides in these tissues is very uncertain.

It is 'common' knowledge that stimulation of sacral nerves produces erection in man and animals (Habib, 1967). This effect, believed to be cholinergic, is however resistant to atropine, which in controlled experiments does not prevent erection in man or monkey (Wagner and Brindley, 1980); neither does the oral intake of propranolol or phenoxybenzamine in normotensive young adults when the compounds have been taken for a few days. These studies were made in controlled situations where erectile capability was recorded. No other quantitative studies of the influence of compounds seem to have been undertaken, although they would be of great value to the clinician.

Recently, one of the peptidergic compounds, VIP (vasoactive intestinal polypeptide), considered to be a neurotransmitter or neuromodulator, has been demonstrated in the penis (Polak et al, 1981; Willis et al, 1981). Also we have demonstrated in recent in vitro studies of smooth muscle from

Clinics in Endocrinology and Metabolism — Vol. 11, No. 3, November 1982.
0300-595X/82/11.03/717 $03.00 © 1982 W. B. Saunders Company Ltd

cavernous bodies of rabbit, monkey and man that VIP has a relaxing effect upon this tissue. Usually VIP is found to induce relaxation of smooth muscle in vitro as well as in vivo in the regions where it is active and VIP receptors can be demonstrated.

Thus proper understanding of the neural control and the associated dysfunctions of these erectile systems is not yet possible. It is noteworthy, however, that our theories of erectile physiology are based mainly on anatomical studies and not on functional experiments, and in general the penis has been a neglected organ during the expansive decades of biological science.

The dominating theory of human penile erection until this decade was initiated by the German anatomist von Ebner (1900), who described the 'pads' or 'cushions' inside the vessels of the penis. These smooth muscle polsters supposedly control flow and pressure transmitted into the cavernous space. The cavernous bodies have to obtain a certain intra-cavernous pressure (minimum about 60 mm Hg) in order to produce the stiffness (rigidity) sufficient for vaginal intromission. In young adults, the intracavernous pressure may be only slightly lower than the brachial systolic pressure (100 to 115 mm Hg) (Metz and Wagner, 1981). This is probably different from the situation inside the spongiose body, where according to clinical observation lower pressures are involved. However, the clinical picture of surgically-induced cavernous-spongiose fistulas in cases of priapism (Ebbehoj, 1975) and the comparable congenital anomalies that lead to erectile failure (Ebbehoj and Wagner, 1979) supports the basic concept that the spongiose body and the paired (and uniformly functional) cavernous bodies have different functions and thus differ in their perfusion rates and regulation through the erectile cycle (Wagner and Green, 1981).

Through the early part of the century the German anatomists discussed at length the mechanism of erection based on microscopic findings. An authorative review of this is found in the monograph by Clara (1956). It seems clear that there was no agreement as to how the deep penile (internal) artery, running inside the cavernous body, supplies the cavernous tissue, or how it could be responsible for a sudden build-up to a high pressure. The demonstration of arterio-venous (a-v) shunts outside the tunica albuginea by Conti (1952) did, however, make it possible to put forward a theory involving a complete relaxation of the Ebner pads and a shut-down of the a-v shunts described by Conti as well as a concomitant reduced outflow from the cavernous body resulting from venous constriction. If the deep dorsal artery is the principal vessel supplying the cavernous body, this would increase the flow (and pressure) into the cavernous space during tumescence. This was the dominant theory until recent years. Several investigators and especially Newman (for review see Newman and Northup, 1981), have challenged the theory, not least on the grounds that the Ebner pads are either age-related or pathological and are found in many other organs of the body. More recent investigations have found none or only few of these previously described 'cushions' (Wagner et al, 1982).

Newman and Northup (1981) propose that arterial dilatation may be sufficient to create the intracavernous pressure necessary for erection. They base this assumption on experiments performed in cadavers where by pudendal artery infusion they have been unable to induce erection and attribute this to 'an easier flow through the dorsal arteries'. This failure may be explained by the very recent demonstration of large shunt vessels leading from the deep artery through the tunica albugenia into the spongiose vessels leading back to the venous system (Wagner et al, 1982). Based on the demonstration of these vessels (Figure 1), visualized by vascular casts, a new theory has been proposed. As the vessels are large and contain a thick muscular coat it is assumed that they have a regulatory function. As the same vascular casts also demonstrated what the anatomists by light microscopy have described as helicine arteries, it would seem obvious to propose the theory that the intracavernous a-v anastomoses leading through the tunica are open when the penis is flaccid. By

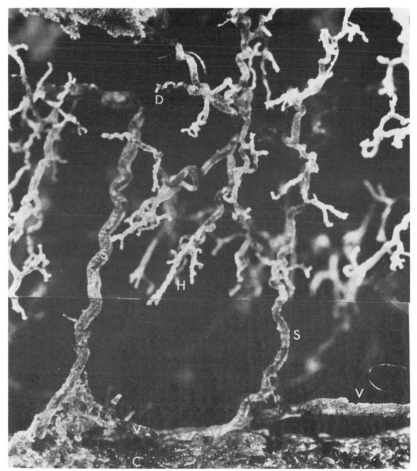

Figure 1. Shunt vessels, visualized by vascular casts, leading from the deep artery through the tunica albugenia (D, deep artery; H, helicine artery, S, shunt vessel; V, vein; C, spongiose body). After Wagner et al (1982), *Lancet,* **ii,** 416-418.

contraction, and thus prevention of run-off from the deep artery, blood flow would be diverted into the helicine arteries that open into the cavernous spaces (Figure 2). Thus this theory involves vasoconstriction, diversion of flow (and pressure) and relaxation of the smooth muscle of the cavernous tissue. Reduced drainage of blood from the cavernous spaces (relative to the maximal outlet) may also be necessary to maintain erection.

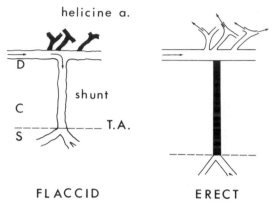

Figure 2. Proposed new theory for the mechanism of erection (see text) (D, deep artery; T.A, tunica albugenia; S, spongiose vessel). (After Wagner et al (1982) *Lancet,* **ii**, 416-418.)

ERECTILE DISORDERS

Abnormal drainage

Wash-out studies, applying the xenon-clearance method (Wagner and Uhrenholdt, 1980), seem to indicate that a sudden decrease in cavernous tissue blood flow rate occurs at the same time as sexual stimulation becomes effective, and that this decrease or very low flow is maintained during sexual stimulation. (For comprehensive discussion of method the reader is referred to Wagner and Green, 1981.) Figure 3 demonstrates an abnormal wash-out, seen in cases where a fistula (or abnormally large, uncontrolled venous drainage) is present. During response to visual sexual stimuli (VSS) tumescence of the penis occurs, but no stiffness, and an increase in outflow is seen (increase in radioactive wash-out from the cavernous body where 200 μCi xenon-133 has been placed before the test). This type of patient will clinically present as having difficulty in maintaining erection for more than a few seconds, often as primary erectile failure as described by Ebbehoj and Wagner (1979) and later confirmed by Virag (1980), Barbe (1981) and Tudoriu (1981).

Besides the xenon wash-out test another clinical diagnostic procedure for the diagnosis of abnormal drainage has been proposed (Virag, 1981). By induced artificial erection, i.e., infusion of normal saline into the cavernous spaces, an erection can be achieved and, once achieved, can be maintained by a much lower infusion rate. The non-anaesthetized patient often will not be aware of the state of his penis and will not be sexually aroused, although

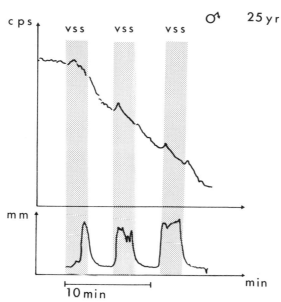

Figure 3. Abnormal wash-out as seen in cases where a fistula (or abnormally large, uncontrolled venous drainage) is present. (VSS = visual sexual stimulation; cps, counts/sec; mm, circumferential change of penis shaft, measured with mercury strain gauge.)

his penis is stiff, and a pressure of 60 mm Hg can be measured. If it is not possible subsequently to reduce the flow (i.e., to about 20 to 30 per cent) whilst maintaining the erection abnormal drainage is suspected. Cavernosography in order to visualize the localization of the defect should be performed, possibly applying the method of infusion cavernosography with simultaneous visual sexual stimulation (Ebbehoj, Uhrenholdt and Wagner, 1980; Wagner and Green, 1981). Surgical intervention with closure of leakages or reducing venous outflow seems to be the treatment method of choice in these cases, though no long-term follow-up studies of such patients have so far been reported.

Priapism

Iatrogenically-induced erectile failure is seen after surgical intervention for priapism. Priapism is a relatively rare condition with permanent erection which eventually becomes painful. Neither its aetiology nor its pathogenesis is understood, though it is seemingly more common among men with sickle cell traits, leukaemia and alcoholism. Priapism may also occur following traumatic events to the perineal region or pelvic fracture. Many cases, however, are not explainable. If untreated, it often leads to fibrosis of the erectile tissue of the corpus cavernosum, which will cause permanent impotence (Money and Hirsch, 1965).

By introduction of a simple, surgical procedure (Ebbehoj, 1975) it has been possible to change the postoperative loss of erection by closure of the induced fistula between the cavernous bodies and the glands. An early surgical intervention is necessary to prevent irreversible damage. If the situation persists for more than 72 hours the prognosis worsens markedly. In a follow-up study of 18 patients Lund and Ebbehoj (1980) found that 11 had normal erectile function, although they had had a surgical fistula induced to terminate the priapism. Another three were rendered potent after closure of the surgically induced fistula. Clearly, those who were in the worst situation were those who had been operated upon late.

A cavernosogram performed during the state of priapism will show no outflow, a situation similar to that seen during full erection in the normal man, indicating that restriction of venous drainage from the cavernous bodies is part of normal erection.

CONCLUSION

Insufficient arterial supply has not been dealt with in this chapter (see Chapter 8), but it should by now be clear that in order to provide rational therapy for the impotent male we require complete understanding of the function of the vessels, their regulation, the nervous pathways, the neurotransmitters and the cerebral connections involved. To reach that ideal goal will need further development of diagnostic and investigative techniques.

REFERENCES

Barbe, A-M. (1981) *Impuissance par Insuffisance Erectile D'Origine Veineuse.* These pour le Doctorat en Medicine. Universite de Paris. 104 pp.

Clara, M. (1956) *Die Arterio-Venosen Anastomosen.* Wien: Springer Verlag. 315 pp.

Conti, G. (1952) L'Erection du penis human et ses basis morphologic-ovasculaires. *Acta Anatomica,* **14,** 217-262.

Ebbehoj, J. (1975) A new operation for priapism. *Scandinavian Journal of Plastic and Reconstructive Surgery,* **8,** 241-242.

Ebbehoj, J. & Wagner, G. (1979) Insufficient penile erection due to abnormal drainage of cavernous bodies. *Urology,* **13,** 507-510.

Ebbehoj, J., Uhrenholdt, A. & Wagner, G. (1980) Infusion cavernosography in the human in the unstimulated and stimulated situations and its diagnostic value. In *Vasculogenic Impotence* (Ed.) Zorgniotti, A. W. & Rossi, G. pp. 191-197. Springfield, Illinois: Charles C. Thomas.

Habib, H. N. (1967) Experimental and recent contribution in sacral nerve stimulation for voiding in both man and animal. *British Journal of Urology,* **39,** 73-83.

Lund, K. & Ebbehoj, J. (1980) Results of glando-cavernous anastomosis in 18 cases of priapism. *Scandinavian Journal of Plastic and Reconstructive Surgery,* **14,** 269-272.

Metz, P. & Wagner, G. (1981) Penile circumference and erection. *Urology,* **18,** 267-270.

Money, J. & Hirsch, S. (1965) After priapism: orgasm retained, erection lost. *Journal of Urology,* **94,** 152-157.

Newman, H. F. & Northup, J. D. (1981) Mechanism of human penile erection: an overview. *Journal of Urology,* **17,** 399-408.

Polak, J. M., Gu, J., Mina, S. & Bloom, S. R. (1981) VIP-ergic nerves in the penis. *Lancet,* **ii,** 217-219.

Tudoriu, Th. (1981) The hemodynamics of erection at the level of the penis. *Presented at the 5th World Congress of Sexology,* Jerusalem.

Virag, R. (1980) Syndrome d'erection instable par insuffisance veineuse. *Presented at the 2nd International Conference on Vascular Impotence,* Monaco.

von Ebner, V. (1900) Uber klappenartige vorrichtungen in der arterien der schwellkorper. *Anatomische Anzeige,* **18,** 79-81.

Wagner, G. & Brindley, G. S. (1980) The effect of atropine, alpha and beta blockers on human penile erections: a controlled pilot study. In *Vasculogenic Impotence* (Ed.) Zorgniotti, A. W. & Rossi, G. pp. 77-81. Springfield, Illinois: Charles C. Thomas.

Wagner, G. & Green, R. (1981) *Impotence, Physiological, Psychological, Surgical Diagnosis and Treatment.* pp. 182. New York, London: Plenum Press.

Wagner, G. & Uhrenholdt, A. (1980) Blood flow measurement by the clearance method in the human corpus cavernosum in the flaccid and erect states. In *Vasculogenic Impotence* (Ed.) Zorgniotti, A. W. & Rossi, G. pp. 41-46. Springfield, Ill: Charles C. Thomas.

Wagner, G. & Uhrenholdt, A. (1982) Blood flow measurement by the clearance method in the human corpus cavernosum in the flaccid and erect states. In *Vasculogenic Impotence, Proceedings of the First International Conference on Corpus Cavernosum Revascularization* (Ed.) Zorgniotti, A. W. & Rossi, G. 1980, pp. 41-46. Springfield, Ill: Charles C. Thomas.

Wagner, G., Bro-Rasmussen, F., Willis, E. A. & Nielsen, M. H. (1982) New theory on the mechanism of erection involving hitherto undescribed vessels. *Lancet,* **ii,** 416-418.

Willis, E., Ottesen, B., Wagner, G., Sundler, F. & Fahrenkrug, J. (1981) Vasoactive intestinal polypeptide (VIP) as a possible neurotransmitter involved in penile erection. *Acta Physiologica Scandinavica,* **13,** 545-547.

8

Arterial Disease as a Cause of Impotence

VÁCLAV MICHAL

INTRODUCTION

Impotence is a disease or a symptom of multiple aetiology which can result from failure of any link in the chain of events leading up to erection. They include the mechanism and haemodynamics of erection, its neurophysiology and hormonal regulation.

Until a few years ago attention was concentrated on the endocrine, nervous and chiefly on psychic factors in the genesis of impotence. Almost no attention was paid to the mechanism and haemodynamics of erection. In recent years the views on the aetiology of impotence in a large portion of patients have been changing. The change in views has given rise to a new term and recognition of a new entity: vasculogenic or angiogenic impotence. Vasculogenic impotence is a failure of the mechanism of erection due either to organic insufficiency of the arterial bed supplying the cavernous bodies — arteriogenic impotence — or to their excessive venous drainage (inadequate blockage of the venous run-off) — which may be called, for want of a more appropriate term, phlebogenic impotence.

ARTERIOGENIC IMPOTENCE

The arterial bed (Figure 1) supplying the cavernous bodies can be divided into two parts. The proximal part is common to the arterial supply of the lower extremities (the aortoiliac area). The distal part, which we called the hypogastricocavernous system (HCS), comprises: the hypogastric (internal iliac) internal pudendal, penile, bulbourethral, dorsal and deep penile arteries and its branches up to the helicoid arteries, terminating in the lacunae of the cavernous bodies. The common denominator of insufficiency of both parts is impairment of erection and impotence, but their symptomatology is different.

Aortoiliac Occlusive Disease

In 1940 Leriche described a syndrome characterized by ischaemia of the lower limbs and by erectile impotence. The pathological basis of this

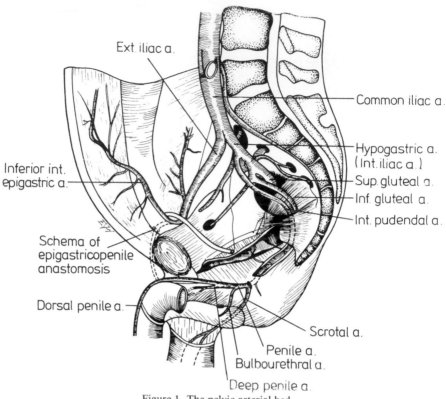

Figure 1. The pelvic arterial bed.

syndrome was occlusion of the aortic bifurcation. It was the first clinical demonstration that arterial occlusion can result in failure of the penis to achieve erection.

In 1958 O'Connor reported a case of Leriche syndrome where endarterectomy of aortic bifurcation resulted also in restoration of sexual activity. In 1960 Scheer expressed the view that not only occlusions of aortic bifurcation but also stenoses and occlusions of the common iliac and hypogastric arteries might cause erectile disorders.

The situation became somewhat more complicated in 1965 when Harris and Jepson reported that aortoiliac reconstruction improved potency in only a small proportion of patients. A larger group complained of worsening and of new development of impotence. Similar results were reported by May, DeWeese and Rob (1969) and other investigators (Spiro and Cotton, 1970). In addition, 50 to 70 per cent of patients undergoing aortoiliac surgery developed ejaculatory disorders (dry emission). Some authors·(Weinstein and Machleder, 1975; De Palma, Levine and Feldman, 1978) attributed both types of sexual disorders to interruption of the preáortic vegetative plexi on dissection of aortic bifurcation. May, De Weese and Rob (1969) held the latter responsible only for the ejaculatory disorders and attributed the worsening of potency to those surgical procedures that decrease arterial flow into the roots of the hypogastric arteries (some of the aortofemoral bypasses). In the seventies this view was confirmed by the studies of Michal et al (1973, 1974, 1976, 1980) and Queral et al (1979).

At present there is sufficient evidence that aortoiliac occlusive disease is associated with erectile disorders in a high number of cases and that their cause is limited flow into the branches of the internal iliac arteries. This postulation is documented by the incidence of erectile disorders, arteriographic findings and decreased blood pressures in the arteries of the penis in patients with aortoiliac disease who complain of impotence and subsequently report restoration or a marked improvement of erectivity after surgery which also restores flow to the branches of the internal iliac arteries.

Estimates of the prevalence of impotence and erectile disorders in aortoiliac occlusive disease vary among authors from 40 to 80 per cent, depending on the definition of impotence and the selection of patient groups. May, De Weese and Rob (1969) report impaired erection in 50 per cent of patients with aortoiliac stenoses and 70 per cent of those with occlusions. Herman, Adar and Rubinstein (1978) describe total impotence in 36 per cent of cases of arteriosclerotic disease of the lower extremities and in 56 per cent if associated with diabetes mellitus. According to our observations (Michal et al, 1973, 1974, 1976, 1980) aortoiliac occlusive disease is associated with impaired erection or impotence in 40 to 50 per cent and 17 to 30 per cent of patients respectively (from the group of patients indicated for aortoiliac surgery, excluding those older than 55 and those with diabetes, rest pain, or gangrene). In about one-third of patients sexual complaints coincide with claudication, but they can also appear several years before or after its onset.

In patients with erectile disorders, the analysis of aortographic findings usually shows bilateral stenoses and occlusions of the arterial pathway up to the branching of the hypogastric arteries. Stenoses or occlusions of the origin of the hypogastric arteries occur in 60 to 80 per cent of these patients.

In the vascular laboratory changes can be detected in the haemodynamic parameters of blood flow in the arteries of the penis. The simplest and commonest test is the measurement of systolic pressure in the penile arteries, which reveals a substantial decrease compared with the brachial artery pressure. A small pressure cuff is placed round the base of the penis. The return of pulsation as systolic pressure is approached can be detected by sensitive plethysmography or by the Doppler ultrasound technique (10 MHz). The latter is the most used and has the following advantages: the pulse in the dorsal and deep penile arteries can be differentiated, and small, simple devices can be used in the office or at the bedside. The values obtained are compared with the systolic pressure in the arm, and the difference between the two is most frequently expressed as a ratio — the *penile-brachial pressure index* (PBPI): PBPI = penile systolic BP/brachial systolic BP.

Recently the following criteria have been adopted by some investigators: PBPI values of less than 0.6 indicate arteriogenic impotence; a value between 0.6 and 0.75 is compatible with the diagnosis but is not diagnostic, while values of greater than 0.75 are considered normal. We should like to point out that these criteria (Gaskell, 1971; Engel, Burnham and Michael, 1978; Queral et al, 1979) were evolved predominantly in groups of patients with aortoiliac stenoses and occlusions and apply to them. As we shall see later, they are not valid for patients with impotence and stenoses or occlusions of the peripheral part of the hypogastricocavernous system. In these patients PBPI can confirm but not exclude arteriogenic impotence (even if equal to or greater than 1.0). Many peripheral stenoses and occlusions that may underlie impotence need not manifest themselves by a decrease of penile systolic pressure at rest (i.e., in the flaccid penis).

Aortoiliac reconstruction, if performed properly, can increase blood flow not only to the lower limbs but also to the pelvic floor, thereby improving or restoring potency in 60 to 80 per cent of the patients (Michal et al, 1973, 1974, 1976, 1980; Virag et al, 1981). Improvement in patients with erectile impairment is taken to mean occurrence of erections sufficient in quality and duration (usually with an increase of coital frequency) and, in patients with complete impotence, restoration of sexual life. Reconstruction fails to improve potency in about 20 per cent of patients. This can be attributed either to postoperative occlusion of the hypogastric arteries or to further peripheral stenoses and occlusions. A criterion can be the postoperative PBPI. A marked improvement in erection was recorded in all patients with a significant postoperative increase of PBPI (Queral et al, 1979; Virag et al, 1981).

Pelvic Steal Syndrome

The first case of a clear steal syndrome in the pelvic area was reported in 1978 (Michal, Kramář and Pospíchal). A 50-year-old patient with occlusion of the right common iliac artery and stenosis of the root of the left hypogastric artery complained of intermittent claudication and erectile insufficiency. He reported achieving and maintaining erection only at rest, with it receding immediately on the start of coital movements. Following aortoiliac reconstruction and endarterectomy of the hypogastric artery, his sexual life normalized and claudication disappeared. Other authors have made similar observations (Métz and Mathiesem, 1979; Querall et al, 1979).

The syndrome is characterized by a change in the distribution of a limited blood flow during loading of the gluteal and femoral muscles. The working muscles 'steal' the blood normally delivered to the cavernous bodies. Nath et al (1981) found that after a gluteal muscle exercise test there was a significant decrease of PBPI in a high portion (38 per cent) of patients examined for erectile disorders. These observations suggest that the steal phenomenon is more frequently implicated in the pathogenesis of erectile insufficiency than hitherto suspected.

Insufficiency of the Hypogastricocavernous System (HCS)

In 1963 Canning et al used impedance plethysmography to evaluate penile blood flow in ten controls and in 41 patients with impotence. In 26 of them they found a flattening of the penile pulse tracing. They concluded that pelvic vascular insufficiency could be a more frequent cause of impotence than previously suspected.

In 1971 Gaskell, using a spectroscopic method, measured blood pressure in the dorsal penile artery in patients with peripheral vascular disease and impotence. He found a marked decrease of pressure in the dorsal penile arteries in a high percentage of patients with impotence, and drew conclusions similar to those of Canning.

Arterial insufficiency of the HCS, assumed by Canning et al (1963), Gaskell (1971) and Michal et al (1973a, 1974) to be present in some patients with impotence, was documented by arteriography in two independent studies in 1976. Ginestié and Romieu (1976) reported stenoses, occlusions and dysplasia of this arterial bed demonstrated by selective arteriography of the hypogastric and internal pudendal arteries. Our technique — a combination of arteriography and artificial erection which we called phalloarteriography — was published the same year and produced similar results (Michal, Pospíchal and Lachman, 1976).

A histological study of the arterial bed of the penis confirmed a high prevalence of stenoses and occlusions in older age groups and in diabetics (Ružbarský and Michal, 1977).

Phalloarteriography

Phalloarteriography (Michal et al, 1976, 1978, 1980) is a selective arteriography of the hypogastricocavernous system during its loading by artificial erection. It allows a good visualization of this arterial bed, including the penile arteries and their branches up to the cavernous bodies (Figure 2).

Artificial erection is induced by infusion of heparinized saline into the cavernous bodies. Under general or local anaesthesia a plastic needle is inserted dorsally into the cavernous body through the preputial insertion just behind the corona of the glans. At the site of puncture the mucosa adheres firmly to the tunica albuginea of the cavernous bodies. There is no bleeding into the subcutaneous tissue after extraction of the needle. The needle is connected to a rotary pump which permits exact regulation and recording of the rate of infusion. The infusion rate is gradually increased until erection is achieved and then reduced to the values sufficient to maintain erection.

Initially we used one infusion line, but now we insert an additional thin plastic needle into the cavernous bodies for measuring intracavernous pressures. An electric manometer is coupled by feedback to the pump to regulate the flow rate. In this way the intracavernous pressure can be maintained at a chosen level and examination can be performed at standard intracavernous pressures of 40 to 50 mm Hg (higher pressures could compress the intracavernous arterial bed).

Continuous recording of intracavernous pressures, infusion rates and changes in the penile circumference yields important diagnostic data as well as some basic information about haemodynamics of erection.

Selective arteriography is performed in both oblique projections by introducing Seldinger catheters into the origins of the hypogastric arteries.

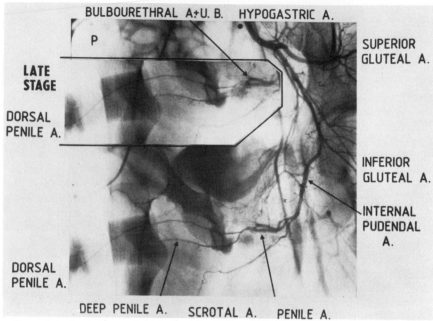

Figure 2. Left-sided normal phalloarteriogram of a 22-year-old patient of the control group.

Until now we have always performed phalloarteriographic examination under general or epidural anaesthesia.

Advantages of a combination of arteriography and artificial erection. A comparative study performed in the same patients both without and with artificial erection showed that the latter induces *selective dilatation* of the peripheral part of the hypogastricocavernous system (Figure 3). The internal pudendal and penile arteries double their diameters in younger individuals. The tortuous course of the arteries straightens and elongates. The enlargement and straightening of the penile arteries minimizes the possibility of overlooking the stenoses which can go undetected under normal conditions. Further advantages of this technique include:

1. The circumference of the erect penis can be measured and can serve as a 100 per cent baseline for measuring nocturnal penile tumescence (NPT).
2. Plastic induration of the penis becomes immediately visible. (Many patients are unaware of the deformation of the penis because they do not achieve erection; some indurations can go unrecognized also on palpation.)
3. The infusion rate needed for achieving and maintaining erection is monitored. High flow rates needed for maintaining erection prove an insufficient blockage of venous run-off and are therefore indicative of phlebogenic impotence.
4. About 20 per cent of our patients reported a distinct improvement in erectile capability lasting several days, weeks, or months following phalloarteriography. The cause of this improvement is not clear.

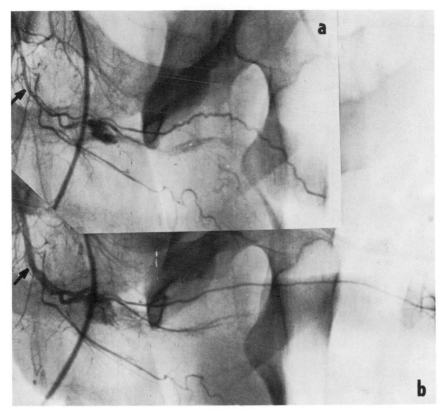

Figure 3. Comparison of the same stages of arteriography without (a) and with (b) artificial erections. Note selective dilatation of the internal pudendal (arrow) and penile arteries (the diameter of the scrotal arteries does not change) and straightening of the latter in erected penis.

Phalloarteriographic findings. Phalloarteriography has demonstrated two types of abnormality of the HCS: occlusions and stenoses, and dysplasia.

Stenoses and occlusions are either of traumatic or of sclerotic origin. Trauma-related lesions have been demonstrated in patients with impotence following pelvic or penile fractures. Occlusions and stenoses were commonly localized in the internal pudendal and penile arteries at the site of the previous fracture of pubic bone (see Figure 6). Three men with a history of penile fractures exhibited homolateral occlusions of the deep penile artery at the site of fracture of the cavernous body. In one of them high flow rate values needed for maintaining erection suggested the presence of a cavernosospongeous fistula, later confirmed by cavernosography.

Stenoses and occlusions (Figure 4) of sclerotic origin occur in diabetics, hypertensives, and men over 36. They have the following pattern:

1. Isolated stenoses and occlusions of the hypogastric and the origin of the internal pudendal arteries.
2. Diffuse changes of the internal pudendal and penile arteries.

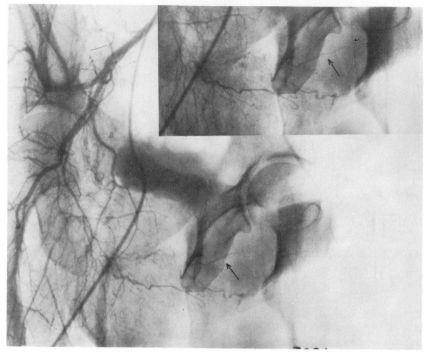

Figure 4. Occlusion of the deep penile, penile and dorsal penile arteries. The periphery of the deep penile artery (arrow) is filled by small collaterals.

3. Involvement of the distal third of the internal pudendal artery, the penile artery and its branches (the most common type).

Dysplasia of the penile arteries (Figure 5) was originally described by Ginestié and Romieu (1976). It involves malformations of the arterial bed of the penis, mainly unilateral or bilateral hypoplasia or aplasia of the deep penile artery. Unilateral severe hypoplasia or aplasia is often associated with hypertrophy of the corresponding contralateral artery. In two of our patients we observed involvement of the penile artery and its branching reminiscent of changes observed mostly in the area of renal arteries and known as fibromuscular hyperplasia.

In addition, a comparison of the phalloarteriographic findings demonstrated high reserves in the capacity and dilatory ability of the HCS in younger individuals which gradually decrease with age even if this arterial bed remains patent. This decrease may be related to prolongation of the time required for achieving erection in higher age groups.

Between 1975 and 1980 phalloarteriography was performed in 248 patients with severe erectile disorders and in 14 males of the control group. The controls comprised three men with normal erectile capability examined by phalloarteriography for haemangiomas in the gluteal and perineal regions, two men with obvious neurogenic impotence (multiple sclerosis),

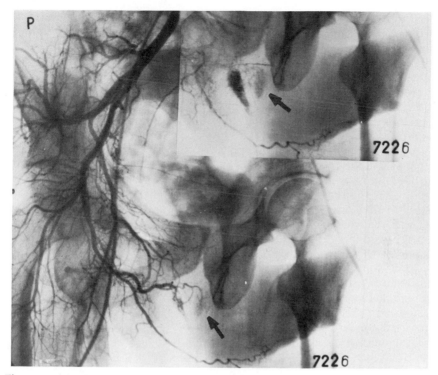

Figure 5. Right-sided phalloarteriogram of dysplasia of the penile arteries. The deep penile artery is hypoplastic and supplies (in the late stage) only a very small area of the cavernous tissue (arrow). The stump of the dorsal penile artery fills only in the late stage and has no outflow (inset). (Primary impotence — 36-year-old patient.)

and nine men, with selective impotence. These nine men reported normal erection in the daytime but failure to achieve an erection with a woman to whom they were attracted most. In the control group phalloarteriography did not show any pathology in the arterial supply of the cavernous bodies. The group of patients was selective since most patients had been referred to us by sexologists or by the Institute of Sexology (Charles University), many after unsuccessful medical treatment and psychotherapy. Arteriographic evidence of insufficiency of the hypogastricocavernous system was established in 186 patients, that is, 76 per cent. (For further details see section entitled 'Arterial basis of organic and psychogenic impotence'.)

HAEMODYNAMIC ASPECTS OF ARTERIOGENIC IMPOTENCE

Erection elicits changes in two basic physical parameters — volume and pressure.

The *basic volume change* is the difference in penile volume between the completely flaccid and fully erect state (erectile volume). It is also the minimal blood volume which the arterial system must supply to achieve full erection. Calculations made from the changes in circumference and length of the penis during erection give a range of the volume change in medium-sized organs between 100 and 140 ml.

The quality of erection can be expressed by a single parameter: *intracavernous pressure*. The measurements we made during artificial erection showed an increase in intracavernous pressure from 15 mm Hg to the levels of mean arterial pressure. At maximum erection during contraction of the ischiocavernous muscles intracavernous pressure reaches suprasystolic values.

During erection the arterial bed must supply the penis at least with minimal volumes of 100 to 140 ml (provided there is no return in venous outflow) and the basic pressure between diastolic and mean arterial pressures. These volumes and pressures can be considered critical or threshold values: if they are not achieved a full erection is impossible.

The aortoiliac bed supplies large muscle areas. Approximately 1 per cent of its rest flow is delivered to the cavernous bodies. The limiting effect of lesions of the aortoiliac area will manifest itself by a decrease in filling pressure for the internal pudendal artery. Only those lesions of the aortoiliac bed that are associated with a pressure gradient and a pressure decrease below the critical values distal to the lesion will affect the haemodynamics of erection. These lesions manifest themselves even at rest by a decreased pressure in the arteries of the penis.

The penile artery supplies exclusively — and the internal pudendal artery almost exclusively — the erectile bodies. Rest flow across the penile arterial bed is estimated at 5 to 10 ml/min or thereabouts (Wagner and Uhrenholdt, 1980; Shiray and Ishii, 1981). Therefore many lesions in the peripheral part of the HCS become haemodynamically significant only at the time of loading by erection. These lesions do not limit rest flow (they are not detectable by PBPI measurement), but they significantly decrease volume delivery during erection. In the first stage they manifest themselves by a substantial prolongation of the filling time of the cavernous bodies, and in the second stage they do so by a decrease in filling pressure.

CLINICAL ASPECTS OF ARTERIAL INSUFFICIENCY

The haemodynamic consequences of restricted blood input to the cavernous bodies are prolongation of the time needed for achieving erection in the initial stage, decreased quality of erection in the second stage, and failure to achieve erection in the late stage.

Prolongation of erectile time

A slight prolongation of erectile time need not have any serious consequences and is well known to the older generation. In contrast with ages between 16 and 30, when minimal erotogenic stimuli suffice to induce an immediate and full response, at ages of about 50 induction of erection requires a longer exposure to intensive erotogenic stimuli, patience, relaxation and time.

A more significant prolongation manifests itself particularly at a time when the patient expects a rapid erection, for example prior to coitus with a new partner. Failure to achieve erection when expected results in psychogenic stress, sympathicotonia and wash-out of adrenergic compounds. On the one hand this raises the patient's blood pressure, on the other vasoconstriction probably further decreases volume delivery to the cavernous bodies and can result in insufficient erection or its complete failure. Repeated experience of this kind induces a whole complex of psychic, emotional and neurovegetative responses known as performance anxiety and psychosexual impotence.

Premature ejaculation. A significant prolongation of the time needed for achieving erection may manifest itself also by interaction with the ejaculation reflex and orgasm. Ejaculation and orgasm are the resultants of the frequency of tactile stimuli from the genital area, the length of exposure to these stimuli and a degree of overall sexual excitement. A significant prolongation automatically leads to intensified psychogenic stimulation but also to tactile stimulation of the organ by the partner in order to induce erection. Intensive stimulation may eventually succeed, but at the same time the interval between achieving erection and ejaculation shortens. This type of premature ejaculation was described by Shapiro 40 years ago.

Incomplete and unsustained erections are the most frequent complaints. A large group of patients with impaired erection report erection after a prolonged intensive stimulation which is, however, followed by immediate ejaculation. Another group complain of disappearance of erection before or without ejaculation. Some of these cases can be explained by the pelvic steal syndrome.

Decrease in quality

Thus far, we have dealt with patients in whom flow, although restricted, is nevertheless sufficient to achieve at least threshold erectile pressures and volumes. Probably many of them can achieve full sleep erections because the duration of vegetative impulses during REM sleep is long enough to induce erection in men with borderline flow restriction. In sleep all stress factors, emerging particularly at the time of imminent coitus, are absent. If inflow is decreased to values below the threshold levels, even maximum stimulation fails to induce sufficient erection and tactile stimulation leads to ejaculation without erection.

ARTERIAL BASIS OF PSYCHOGENIC AND ORGANIC IMPOTENCE

Traditional concepts subdivide the pathological causes of impotence into organic (where impotence is one symptom of another disease or posttraumatic state) and psychogenic (where impotence is the disease and has psychological causes) — see Table 1. It is estimated and generally accepted that 90 per cent of all cases are psychogenic, so that an organic basis should exist in only 10 per cent of cases.

Organic Impotence

In Table 1 the group of organic diseases is further subdivided according to the clear and unclear relationships of impotence to the primary disease. The

Table 1. *Traditional subdivision of impotence*

Organic impotence (10%)

Causality :	Relatively clear	Unclear (most frequent)
	neurogenic	hypertension
	androgenic	diabetes mellitus
	pharmacogenic	peripheral arteriosclerosis
	aortoiliac disease	myocardial infarction
	genitourinary diseases	ischaemic heart disease

Psychogenic impotence (90%)

primary — rare
constitutional — relatively rare
secondary (acquired) — most frequent

group of unclear pathogenesis comprises by far the most frequent organic causes of impotence, namely diabetes, states after myocardial infarction and ischaemic heart disease, hypertension and peripheral atherosclerosis. The pathogenesis of these organic causes is a matter of speculation, unproved theory and often related to psychological factors. However, these diseases have in common one more, hitherto ignored, factor — they are either diseases of other parts of the arterial system or they are, according to epidemiological evidence, high risk factors of arterial diseases in general.

In 86 patients examined phalloarteriographically impotence was related to a disease or posttraumatic state that falls into the category of the organic causes of impotence (Table 2).

Table 2. *Phalloarteriographic results in patients with organic impotence*

Primary disease	No.	HCS lesions	%	Contributing factors
Myocardial infarction (MI)				
+ ischaemic heart disease (IHD)	9	9	100.0	
Peripheral arteriosclerosis	11	11	100.0	
Diabetes mellitus (DM)	34	33	97.1	neuropathy
Hypertension	17	11	64.7	pharmacogenic
Pelvic fractures	12	12	100.0	
Penile fractures	3	3	100.0	phlebogenic
Total	86	79	92.0	

Plastic induration in 24% of HCS stenoses and occlusions, 0.3—0.03% in normal population

Myocardial infarction (MI) and ischaemic heart disease (IHD)

It has been known since 1964 that two thirds to three quarters of the patients after MI report severe erectile disorders or 'sexual abstinence' (Tuttle, Cook and Fitch, 1964; Klein et al, 1965). Until 1980 impotence in postinfarction patients was considered to be a consequence of the psychological reaction to the MI (performance anxiety resulting from fear of bodily motion, reinfarction or death). In 1980 two publications appeared almost simultaneously, both with the same message: not only do sexual problems arise for the male after infarction but in 50 to 70 per cent of men they also preceded the infarction. Wabrek and Burchell investigated 131 males during hospitalization for acute MI. Zvěřina and Raboch examined 118 males during spa treatment three to six months after the episode. Both of these groups of authors expressed the similar view that an unsuccessful sex life before the MI can be both cause and result of psychological tension which becomes a causative factor for the MI itself.

In our outpatient clinic we examined for inadequate erection 20 patients with IHD of whom ten sustained MI. In only three of the ten patients did the onset of the sexual difficulties fall within a five-month period following the acute MI. After cardiological and anaesthesiological consultation we carried out phalloarteriography in nine of the 20 IHD patients. In all of them examination showed stenoses and occlusions of HCS.

These observations show that sexual problems in patients with ischaemic heart disease represent a coexistence of involvement of yet another vascular bed, both with the same occlusive disease.

Manifest peripheral arteriosclerosis

Eleven of our total group of patients subjected to phalloarteriography also showed signs of arteriosclerotic occlusions and narrowings in the peripheral vascular bed. This group does not include any patients with IHD or aorto-iliac occlusion. The group of 11 reported either intermittent claudication of moderate degree (walking distance over 500 m) or reported only feeling 'tired in their legs'. In all 11, phalloarteriography showed occlusions or narrowings in the hypogastricocavernous arterial axis.

Diabetes mellitus (DM)

The role of vascular factors in the pathogenesis of impotence in diabetics has in the past been mainly speculative in nature, taking origin from the existence of diabetic angiopathy (mainly affecting the microcirculation) and the generally accepted susceptibility of diabetics to vascular, mainly arteriosclerotic, disease.

In 1971 Gaskell reported a significant decrease in systolic blood pressure in the dorsal penile artery in seven of eight impotent patients hospitalized for peripheral vascular occlusions in diabetes. In 1975 Abelson measured pressure in the dorsal penile artery in 15 impotent diabetics by the Doppler ultrasound technique. In only six could he find decreases in systolic pressure which would suggest a flow block in the inflow channels.

Michal, Pospíchal and Lachman (1976) reported on 12 patients with diabetic impotence, investigated by phalloarteriography. In all patients they found narrowings and occlusions in the hypogastricocavernous inflow paths. In 1977 they reported on a histological study of the arterial bed of the penis in 15 diabetics and 15 control males dying of other causes. This study showed that pathological changes limiting inflow of blood into the cavernous bodies were, age group for age group, far more severe in the diabetic population (Ružbarský and Michal, 1977).

In 1975 to 1980 we investigated by phalloarteriography 34 patients with erectile inadequacy and DM. Four patients fell into the juvenile diabetic group with ages of onset 12, 14, 17 and 18 years. Erectile abnormalities in these patients occurred at age 22 in two and between 34 and 37 years of age in the other two. All four were impotent. Nine of the group (26.4 per cent) had clinical and case history evidence of arterial disease outside of the aortoiliac region (narrowing or occlusion of the arteries of the lower extremity distal to the common femoral artery, or ischaemic heart disease). One patient had suffered a slight case of brain ischaemia with residua of hemiparesis. Sixteen males with incomplete and short-lasting erections reported a decrease in coital frequency to one sixth of starting levels (on an average four years from the start of erectile difficulties). Eighteen males were impotent. It is of interest that none of the patients reported complete night erections.

We could find no correlation between the degree of erectile difficulties and their duration, nor with the duration and severity of the DM, treatment of the DM, or involvement with other regions of the arterial bed.

In all patients with diabetic erectile difficulties phalloarteriography showed narrowing and occlusions of the vascular bed supplying blood to the cavernous bodies. Only in one case was it possible to doubt the haemo-dynamic significance of a clear occlusion of the deep penile artery bridged by a wide collateral. We used a simple system of classifying these changes: 1, severe narrowing of one hypogastricocavernous pathway; 2, unilateral occlusion; no changes on either side was rated as 0, and bilateral occlusions were rated as 4. This system was found to be of use even if a certain degree of subjectivity in analysing the x-ray changes played a role. This numerical evaluation was found to agree well with both complaints and clinical observations. The mean rating in the group of impotent patients was 3.5 ± 1.2 and 2.7 ± 0.9 in patients with incomplete and short-lasting erections.

Our results show some discrepancy with those of Abelson (1975) who reported a significant decrease in penile arterial pressure in only six (40 per cent) of 15 cases of diabetic impotence. It is suggested that this discrepancy is due to the fact that neither narrowing nor occlusions of the internal pudendal and penile arteries, and even to a lesser degree changes in the deep penile artery, need be reflected in significant decreases in pressure measured in the dorsal penile artery at rest. On the other hand, Karacan, Salis and Williams (1978) measured blood pressure in the dorsal penile artery in 12 diabetics who did not achieve full erection at NPT and found a decrease of PBPI to the mean value 0.58 (58 per cent of brachial pressure).

Five of our patients reported a disappearance of ejaculation. These findings reflect abnormal regulation of the ejaculation reflex which suggest that neuropathy exists in the region of the pelvic autonomic plexi (reported in 1971 by Ellenberg). Twelve of the patients (Lachman et al, 1976) were investigated by cystometry. Eight of them (66 per cent) showed pathological cystometrograms, which suggests neuropathology in this innervation as well. It would appear, therefore, that two components play a role in the development of diabetic impotence: limitation of the blood flow into the cavernous bodies by narrowings and occlusion of the hypogastrico-cavernous pathway, and diabetic neuropathy in the autonomic pelvic plexi. Only further observation, especially the results of revascularization procedures, can delimit what fractional importance can be attached to each factor category.

Hypertension

Stenoses and occlusions of HCS were present only in 65 per cent of hypertensive patients with erectile disorders. A pharmacogenic component due to antihypertensive therapy with drugs containing reserpine, methyldopa and quanethidine was probably also involved.

Pelvic fractures

These have already been dealt with in the section entitled 'Phalloarteriographic findings'.

Induratio penis plastica (Peyronie's disease)

The first 30 phalloarteriographies performed in our clinic revealed a fairly high incidence of plastic induration of the penis in patients with erectile inadequacy who also showed narrowings and occlusions of the hypogastrico-cavernous vascular pathway (Michal and Pospíchal, 1978). Of the total number of 156 stenoses and occlusions, plastic induration of the penis (Peyronie's disease) was established in 39 (24 per cent of cases). Its prevalence in the normal population is estimated at 0.3 (Tuffier, 1885) to 0.03 per cent (Polkey, 1928). The high prevalence in our series as well as clinical observations suggest that ischaemic changes, primarily in the tributary of the dorsal penile artery, play a role in the pathogenesis of Peyronie's disease.

'Psychogenic' Impotence

Our group comprises 158 phalloarteriographically examined patients with impotence which would be routinely classified as psychogenic. Using standard criteria, we divided them into three groups — primary, constitutional, and secondary (i.e., acquired impotence).

Primary and constitutional impotence

The first two groups are composed of men who have never experienced sexual intercourse and men who have always had difficulties in achieving and maintaining erection and report low coital frequency, usually below 50 per year. (See Table 3.)

The average age of the group of 26 patients with primary impotence was 25.4 ± 5.2. Two of this group reported that they had never experienced an erection; the remaining 24 reported incomplete erection, insufficient for coitus, and 16 of these reported in addition that the incomplete erection was also transitory. Usually they experienced ejaculation with an erection inadequate for penetration.

Table 3. *Phalloarteriographic findings in 'psychogenic' impotence*

'Psychogenic' impotence	Average age	No.	Finding: dysplasia	%
Primary	25.4	26	16	61.5
Constitutional	28.5	16	11	68.7
Total	26.6	42	27	64.3
Secondary (acquired)			stenoses + occlusions	
Age < 35 years	34.1	28	2	7.1
Age > 35 years	48.2	88	78	88.6
Total	40.0	158	107	67.7

The group of constitutional impotence comprised 16 men. Coital frequency before the acute worsening which brought the patient to our clinic averaged 37 per year despite the fact that the mean age was 28.5 ± 4.1. In the year previous to admission this mean value had decreased to nil in nine patients and to a mean value of 9.5 (range 1 to 18). None of the above patients reported complete absence of erection, rather they complained of weak erection of short duration.

Phalloarteriography demonstrated arterial dysplasia of the penis in 27 (64.3 per cent) cases out of 42 investigations for primary and constitutional impotence. These findings suggest that developmental abnormalities of the arterial bed of the penis play an important, if not critical, role in the pathogenesis of both types of impotence in a large group of patients.

Primary impotence has been attributed to psychic trauma in childhood and adolescence, religious orthodoxy, Oedipus complex, traumatic experience with prostitutes, alcoholism, traumatic experience at first coitus, and to the unexplained sensitivity to psychosocial factors (Masters and Johnson, 1970). In agreement with the observations of Ginestié and Romieu (1976) and on the basis of our findings it can be argued that in a number of cases this unexplained sensitivity in primary impotence is a developmental abnormality of the arterial supply to the cavernous bodies.

Phalloarteriography shows that arteriogenic impotence, either primary or constitutional in nature, has a constant bottom line: dysplasia of the arterial bed supplying the penis. Therefore the two groups probably differ only by the degree of affection of the arterial bed and can be modified by psychogenic factors. However, in five cases high flow rates needed for maintaining erection suggest that insufficient blockage of the venous run-off can be also involved (confirmed in two by cavernosography and in three by operation).

Phalloarteriography did not explain ten (23.8 per cent) out of 42 patients with primary and constitutional impotence.

Secondary (acquired) impotence

In connection with organic impotence we have dealt with some risk factors of arterial disease without mentioning the basic one — aging. Thirty-five is the age after which both the incidence of impotence and the incidence of arterial diseases rise rapidly. We have therefore divided the group of secondary impotence into cases with the onset of impotence before and after the age of 35.

Lower age group. The first group includes 28 subjects of mean age 31 ± 4.1 at the time that erectile difficulties arose. At the time of investigation the mean age was 34.1 (the mean duration of erectile difficulties was 3.1 years). The mean coital frequency before the onset of these complaints was 141.4 per year. Only three subjects reported no erections at all. The remaining 25 complained of incomplete and short-lasting erections, and in 13 of these erection was not sufficient to penetrate.

Phalloarteriography showed a normal picture in 26 (92.9 per cent). In two cases there was obliteration of the penile artery bridged by a collateral, in both cases from the region of the obturator artery. In three cases the high levels of flow needed to maintain an artificial erection gave rise to suspicion of abnormal venous drainage of the penis.

Phalloarteriography in subjects with secondary impotence in whom erectile difficulties arose before age 35 suggested that vascular aetiology played a role only in a minority of cases. In the majority of these patients the real cause of impotence remained unknown.

Higher age group. In 88 patients of this series erectile difficulties arose after the age of 36 (mean age of this subgroup was 48.2 ± 6.0). Of these 40 (45.4 per cent) did not attain a sufficient degree of erection to allow coitus (17 reported no erection at all) and 48 (54.6 per cent) complained of incomplete erection which occasionally was sufficient for coitus (this group had shown a decrease in coital frequency from 131 to 20.5 per year).

Phalloarteriography in ten cases (11.4 per cent) showed a generally normal picture of the hypogastricocavernous system bilaterally (i.e., no stenoses exceeding 50 per cent of the lumen). In the remaining cases (88.6 per cent) there were stenoses and occlusions in this bed.

If we use the same classification as in the group of diabetics, then the mean grading of the arterial disease in the whole group would be 2.4 (3.0 ± 0.65 for patients with impotence, 2.1 ± 0.94 for those with weak and short-lasting erection).

It was of interest that flow levels required to maintain an artificial erection exceeded 100 ml/min in 37 cases. Such values were also measured in patients with significant bilateral penile arterial disease. This suggests that a decrease in blood outflow from the cavernous bodies during erection is a function of either age or limitation of arterial inflow, which also suggest that the two flows may be functionally interrelated.

The high percentage of lesions of the hypogastricocavernous system in the older age group compared with the exponential rise of impotence with age reported by Kinsey, Pomeroy and Martin (1948) shows that arteriogenic impotence represents by far the most common type.

Our phalloarteriographic data are in sharp contrast with the usually stated view that 90 per cent of all impotence is of psychogenic origin. For this reason let us try to determine how this latter view came about and what diagnostic criteria were used. The diagnosis of psychogenic impotence is based upon:

1. Exclusion of organic disease which could be associated with impotence.
2. History of spontaneous, mainly night and morning, erections.
3. History underlying the psychic causes of impotence.

Comment on 1. The elimination of organic causes neither rules out nor confirms the psychogenic origin of impotence. It is a proof, if anything, that the cause is unknown, NOT that organic disease is not involved.

Comment on 2. As shown by the steal syndrome, the presence of full erections, no matter how objective the criteria for their determination are, may not exclude an arteriogenic cause. The presence of night and morning erections suggests only a partial role for the psychological component. Prolonged erection time, which is of no consequence in night and morning erections, will also play a role. Objective recording of NPT carried out in an adequate number of subjects shows that 60 per cent of impotent men do not achieve full erection — a further argument against psychogenic aetiology (Karacan, Salis and Williams, 1978; Kaya, Moore and Karacan, 1979).

Comment on 3. The anamnestic findings of conscious or unconscious motives underlying impotence depend on the interpretation of a number of life events by the investigator and the investigated. It is difficult to decide whether the psychic and behavioural moments play a primary or secondary role, and whether they are the cause or result of impotence.

Judging by our observations, we hold that the psychic factor in the pathogenesis of impotence has been overrated. It would certainly be a mistake to underestimate it. If the capacity of the arterial bed supplying the cavernous bodies is limited to values close to and above the critical level, the psychogenic component can play a very important role. In such cases, appropriate psychotherapy, particularly the elimination of psychogenic stress and performance anxiety, can produce and often does produce good results. However, if the arterial bed cannot deliver sufficient volume and pressure to the cavernous bodies, psychosexual therapy, no matter how good it may be, is not capable of improving the state substantially until inflow capacity to the cavernous bodies is increased.

THERAPY OF ARTERIOGENIC IMPOTENCE

Primary, constitutional and posttraumatic arteriogenic impotence is a result of localized arterial involvement, and therapy can be aimed only at improvement and restoration of potency. On the other hand, acquired arteriogenic impotence is one and often the first of the symptoms of a more or less generalized arterial disease. Therapy should be directed primarily at this disease to prevent even more serious complications such as intermittent claudication and gangrene, cerebrovascular disease and stroke or IHD and MI. The importance of the fact that MI is preceded by erectile disorders in 50 to 70 per cent of patients (Wabrek and Burchell, 1980; Zvěřina and Raboch, 1980) should not be underestimated.

Therefore rational *conservative therapy* of acquired arteriogenic impotence should prevent or minimize further progress of arteriosclerosis and eliminate or bring under control all high risk factors of arterial disease. Prohibition of smoking, antisclerotic diet, regular control and therapy of diabetes and hypertension are the first and most important therapeutical measures. They should be applied no matter whether impotence is to be treated by arterial reconstruction, penile implant, psychotherapy, medical therapy, or will remain untreated.

Pharmacotherapy of impotence includes aphrodisiacs, primarily yohimbine, and CNS stimulants (strychnine and extract of nuci vomicae), often in combination with androgens, gonadotrophic hormones and LHRH. The effectiveness of this therapy in patients without clinical and laboratory symptoms of hormonal deficiency, as well as the effectiveness of psychotherapy, could be questioned. The situation was recently summarized by Cooper (1978) as follows: 'A representative sample of the literature on the treatment and prognosis of male potency disorders (e.g., impotence, impotentia ejaculandi, premature ejaculation) is presented: despite the enormous volume of opinion, the amount of reviewable hard data is desultory.'

Surgical treatment consists of revascularization or implantation of different types of penile prostheses.

Revascularization procedures are designed to renew and increase arterial flow to the cavernous bodies. They include reconstruction of the hypogastric and internal pudendal arteries and also microvascular procedures, bypassing the whole proximal part of the HCS — anastomoses of the inferior epigastric artery to the dorsal or deep penile arteries or directly to the cavernous bodies (see Figures 6 and 7). Instead of the epigastric artery some authors use also venous bypasses originating from the common femoral artery. The procedures are part of a newly developing field of vascular surgery. The results of the procedures, indicated on the basis of arteriographic findings, show restoration or improvement of erection in 80 to 90 per cent of reconstructions of the proximal part of the HCS (hypogastric and proximal part of the internal pudendal artery) and in 60 to 80 per cent of reconstructions of the penile arteries and their branches. The basic advantage of these surgical procedures is the restoration of natural erections.

Implantation of penile prosthesis is another surgical solution. Penile implants can insure penetration and some of them can also imitate the function of the cavernous bodies. In arteriogenic impotence they should be indicated only in cases where successful arterial reconstruction is improbable due to the type of involvement of the arterial bed and/or to other contributing factors which may play a major role.

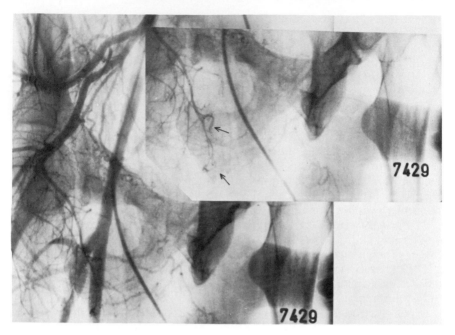

Figure 6. Right-sided phalloarteriogram of a young patient with impotence following bilateral pelvic fracture. In the late stage (right upper corner) note occlusion of the penile and scrotal arteries (arrows) at the site of a previous fracture of the pubic bone. The dorsal and partially also the deep penile arteries are filled via small collaterals.

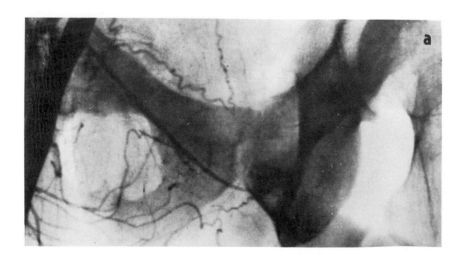

Figure 7(a).

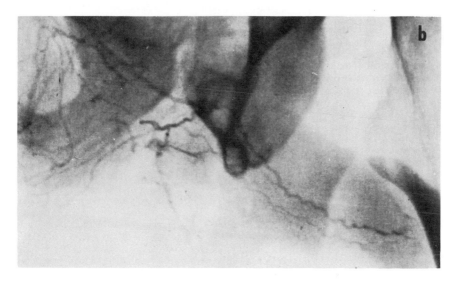

Figure 7. Early (a) and middle (b) stage of control arteriography of an epigastricopenile anastomosis performed in the previous patient (Figure 6) one year after operation. Note filling of the dorsal, deep and accessory deep penile arteries across the anastomosis (b).

SUMMARY

The traditional views on the aetiology of impotence, attributing more than 90 per cent of all cases of impotence to psychic pathogenesis, have changed. Measurement of penile blood pressure, nocturnal penile tumescence studies (NPT) and especially new techniques of arteriographic examination of the arterial bed supplying the cavernous bodies have shown that the majority of cases have an organic basis affecting the haemodynamics of erection (limitation of arterial inflow into the cavernous bodies and/or their excessive venous drainage).

Arterial disease, which is the most frequent affection in the middle-aged and elderly male population, is also largely implicated in the pathogenesis and aetiology of impotence. Recognition of this role of arterial disease is important not only with respect to the treatment of impotence but above all with respect to prevention of even more serious complications of the former condition such as IHD and MI, cerebrovascular disease and stroke, or intermittent claudication and gangrene.

ENDNOTE

Some parts of the text and documentation from the manuscript 'Role of Vascular Disease in Impotence' to be published by Charles C. Thomas: Springfield, Il, USA, were used for this chapter.

REFERENCES

Abelson, D. (1975) Diagnostic value of penile pulse and blood pressure: Doppler study of impotence in diabetics. *Journal of Urology*, 133, 636.

Canning, J. R., Bowers, L. M., Lloyd, F. A. & Cottrell, T. L. C. (1963) Genital vascular insufficiency and potence. *Surgical Forum*, 14, 298.

Cooper, A. J. (1978) Treatment of male potency disorders: the present status. In *Handbook of Sex Therapy* (Ed.) LoPiccolo, J. & LoPiccolo, L. pp. 323-336. New York: Plenum Press.

Crespo, E., Bove, D., Farrell, G. & Soltanik, E. (1980) Tratamiento de la impotencia sexual masculina de causa vascular por revascularización del Pene. *La Prensa Médica*, 67, (15).

DePalma, R. G., Levine, S. B. & Feldman, S. (1978) Preservation of erectile function after aortoiliac reconstruction. *Archives of Surgery*, 113, 958-962.

Ellenberg, M. (1971) Impotence in diabetes: the neurologic factor. *Annals of Internal Medicine*, 75, 213-219.

Engel, G., Burnham, S. J. & Michael, F. C. (1978) Penile blood pressure in the evaluation of erectile impotence. *Fertility and Sterility*, 30, 687-690.

Gaskell, P. (1971) The importance of penile blood pressure in cases of impotence. *Canadian Medical Association Journal*, 105, 1047.

Ginestié, J. F. & Romieu, A. (1976) *L'exploration Radiologique de L'impuissance*. Paris: Maloine. 129 pp. (English translation: *Radiologic Exploration of Impotence* (1978). The Hague: Martinus Nijhoff Medical Division).

Harris, J. D. & Jepson, R. P. (1965) Aortoiliac stenosis: a comparison of two procedures. *Australian and New Zealand Journal of Surgery*, 34, 211-214.

Hermann, A., Adar, R. & Rubinstein, Z. (1978) Vascular lesions associated with impotence in diabetic and nondiabetic arterial occlusive disease. *Diabetes*, 27, 975-981.

Karacan, L. (1980) Diagnosis of erectile impotence in diabetes mellitus. An objective and specific method. *Annals of Internal Medicine*, 92, 334-337.

Karacan, I., Salis, P. J. & Williams, R. L. (1978) The role of the sleep laboratory in diagnosis and treatment of impotence. In *Sleep Disorders. Diagnosis and Treatment* (Ed.) Williams, R. L. & Karacan, I. pp. 358-382. New York: John Wiley.

Kinsey, A. C., Pomeroy, W. B. & Martin, C. E. (1948) *Sexual Behaviour in the Human Male*. pp. 804. Philadelphia: W. B. Saunders.

Klein, R. F., Dean, A., Willson, L. M. & Bogdonoff, M. D. (1965) The physician and post myocardial infarction invalidism. *Journal of the American Medical Association*, 194, 143-148.

Kaya, N., Moore, C. & Karacan, I. (1979) Nocturnal penile tumescence and its role in impotence. *Psychiatric Annals*, 9, 63-68.

Lachman, M., Raboch, J., Michal, V., Pospíchal, J., Bernát, M., Stárka, L., Vomáčka, V. & Vacek, J. (1976) A contribution to the *Pathogenesis of Erectivity Disorders in Diabetics* (in Czech, English summary). *Časopis Lékařů českých*, 115, 1242-1245.

Leriche, R. (1940) De la résection du carrefour aorticoiliaque avec double sympathectomic lombaire pour thrombose arteritique de l'aorte; le syndrome de l'oblitération termino-aortique par artérite. *Press Mèdicale*, 48, 601-604.

Masters, W. H. & Johnson, V. E. (1970) *Human Sexual Inadequacy*. London: Churchill Livingstone.

May, A. G., De Weese, J. A. & Rob, C. E. (1969) Changes in sexual function following operation on the abdominal aorta. *Surgery*, 65, 41.

Metz, P. & Mathiesem, F. R. (1979) External iliac 'steal syndrome' leading to a defect in penile erection and impotence: a case report. *Vascular Surgery*, 13, 70-72.

Michal, V. & Pospíchal, J. (1978) Phalloarteriography in the diagnosis of erectile impotence. *World Journal of Surgery*, 2, 239-247.

Michal, V. & Ružbarský, V. (1980) Histological changes in the penile arterial bed with aging and diabetes. In *Vasculogenic Impotence. Proceedings of the First International Conference on Corpus Cavernosum Revascularization* (Ed.) Zorgniotti, A. W. & Rossi, G. pp. 113-119. Springfield: Charles C. Thomas.

Michal, V., Kramář, R. & Barták, V. (1974) Femoro-pudendal by-pass in the treatment of sexual impotence. *Journal of Cardiovascular Surgery*, 15, 356-359.

Michal, V., Kramář, R. & Hejhal, L. (1980) Revascularization procedures of the cavernous bodies. In *Vasculogenic Impotence. Proceedings of the First International Conference on*

Corpus Cavernosum Revascularization (Ed.) Zorgniotti, A. W. & Rossi, G. pp. 239-255. Springfield: Charles C. Thomas.

Michal, V., Kramář, R. & Pospíchal, J. (1973) Femoro-pudendal by-pass and internal iliac thromboendarterectomy in the treatment of erectile impotence. *Bulletin de la Société Internationale de Chirurgie,* **32,** 387.

Michal, V., Kramář, R. & Pospíchal, J. (1974) Femoro-pudendal by-pass, internal iliac thrombo-endarterectomy and direct arterial anastomosis to the cavernous body in the treatment of erectile impotence. *Bulletin de la Société Internationale de Chirurgie,* **33,** 343-350.

Michal, V., Pospíchal, J. Blažková, J. (1980) Arteriography of the internal pudendal arteries and passive erection. In *Vasculogenic Impotence. Proceedings of the First International Conference on Corpus Cavernosum Revascularization* (Ed.) Zorgniotti, A. W. & Rossi, G. pp. 169-179. Springfield: Charles C. Thomas.

Michal, V., Pospíchal, J. & Lachman, M. (1976) Penile arteries occlusions in erectile impotence. A new type of angiography — phalloarteriography (in Czech, English Summary). *Časopis Lékařů českých,* **115,** 1245-1247.

Michal, V., Kramář, R. & Pospíchal, J. (1978) External iliac 'steal syndrome'. *Journal of Cardiovascular Surgery,* **12,** 355-357.

Michal, V., Kramář, R., Hejhal, L., Firt, P., Hejnal, J. & Barták, V. (1973a) The tactics of reconstruction interventions in aortoiliac area in view of disorders of erectivity in men (in Czech, English summary). *Rozhledy v Chirurgii,* **52,** 591-595.

Michal, V., Kramář, R., Pospíchal, J. & Hejhal, L. (1973b) Direct arterial anastomosis on corpora cavernosa penis in the therapy of erective impotence (in Czech, English Summary). *Rozhledy v Chirurgii,* **52,** 587-590.

Michal, V., Kramář, R., Pospíchal, J. & Hejhal, L. (1976) Gefässchirurgie erektiver impotenz. *Sexualmedizin,* **5,** 15-16 and 20.

Michal, V., Kramář, R., Pospíchal, J. & Hejhal, L. (1977) Arterial epigastrico-cavernous anastomosis for the treatment of sexual impotence. *World Journal of Surgery,* **1,** 515-520.

Michal, V., Kramář, R., Hejhal, L. & Firt, P. (1980) Aortoiliac occlusive disease. In *Vasculogenic Impotence. Proceedings of the First International Conference on Corpus Cavernosum Revascularization* (Ed.) Zorgniotti, A. W. & Rossi, G. pp. 203-215. Springfield: Charles C. Thomas.

Nath, R. L., Menzoian, J. O., Kaplan, K. H., McMillian, T. N., Siroky, M. B. & Krane, K. J. (1981) The multidisciplinary approach to vasculogenic impotence. *Surgery,* **89,** 124-133.

O'Connor, V. J. (1958) Impotence and the Leriche syndrome. An early diagnostic sign, consideration of the mechanism, relief by endarterectomy. *Journal of Urology,* **80,** 195.

Polkey, H. J. (1928) Induratio penis plastica. *Urologic and Cutaneous Review,* **30,** 287.

Queral, L. A., Whitehouse, W. M., Flinn, W. R., Zarins, C. K., Bergan, J. J. & Yao, J. S. T. (1979) Pelvic hemodynamics after aortoiliac reconstruction. *Surgery,* **86,** 799-809.

Ružbarský, V. & Michal, V. (1977) Morphologic changes in the arterial bed of the penis with aging. Relationship to the pathogenesis of impotence. *Investigative Urology,* **15,** 194-199.

Scheer, A. (1960) Die Impotenz als Symptom der arteriellen Durchblutungsstörungen im Beckenbereich. *Münchener Medizinische Wochenschrift,* **36,** 1713-1715.

Shapiro, B. (1943) Premature ejaculation, review of 1130 cases. *Journal of Urology,* **50,** 374-379.

Shiray, M. & Ishii, N. (1981) Haemodynamics of erection in man. *Archives of Andrology,* **6,** 27-32.

Spiro, M. & Cotton, L. T. (1970) Aorto-iliac thromboendarterectomy. *British Journal of Surgery,* **57,** 161-168.

Tuffier, M. (1885) Sur l'induration des corps caverneux. *Archives des Maladies des Reins et des Organs Génito-urinaires,* **3,** 401.

Tuttle, W. B., Cook, W. L. & Fitch, E. (1964) Sexual behaviour in postmyocardial infarction patients. *American Journal of Cardiology,* **13,** 140-143.

Virag, R. (1980) L'exploration Doppler de l'impuissance. Une étude statistique de 103 cas avec 65 controles artériographiques. *Angéiologie,* **33,** 115-122.

Virag, R., Frydman, D., Cadre, N., Legman, M. & Penven, J. P. (1981) Hémodynamique de la circulation artérielle pénienne. Avant et après reconstruction aortoilliaque pour artériopathie oblitérante des membres inférieurs. *Angéiologie,* **33,** 269-274.

Wabrek, A. J. & Burchell, R. C. (1980) Male sexual dysfunction associated with coronary heart disease. *Archives of Sexual Behavior,* **9,** 69-75.

Wagner, G. & Uhrenholdt, A. (1980) Blood flow measurement by the clearance method in the human corpus cavernosum in the flaccid and erect states. In *Vasculogenic Impotence. Proceedings of the First International Conference on Corpus Cavernosum Revascularization* (Ed.) Zorgniotti, A. W. & Rossi, G. pp. 41-46. Springfield: Charles C. Thomas.

Weinstein, M. H. & Machleder, J. I. (1975) Sexual function after aortoiliac surgery. *Annals of Surgery,* **181,** 787-790.

Zvěřina, J. & Raboch, J. (1980) Vorboten des Infarkts. *Sexualmedizin,* **9,** 446-447.

9

The Effects of Diabetes on Male Sexual Function

CHRISTOPHER G. FAIRBURN
DAVID K. McCULLOCH
F. C. WU

INTRODUCTION

Many physical conditions have adverse effects on sexual function. There is usually an obvious relationship between the nature and degree of disability and the type of sexual problem. In diabetes, however, while sexual problems are common among those who are severely handicapped by the disease, they are also found in those patients whose metabolic disturbance is relatively mild and who are otherwise leading an unrestricted life.

The first part of this chapter will describe the various forms of sexual disturbance found among male diabetics. This will be followed by an examination of aetiological factors, and finally consideration will be given to assessment and management. Throughout the chapter the importance of the interplay between physical and psychological factors will be emphasized.

CLINICAL FEATURES

Diabetic patients are subject to two major types of sexual problem. The first is characterized by a reduction in sexual appetite and a degree of erectile failure, both of which may be attributed to the lethargy, tiredness and malaise associated with hyperglycaemia (Kolodny, Masters and Johnson, 1979). This type of sexual disorder is not specific to diabetes, but is found in other debilitating conditions. It may occur at the onset of the disease and during subsequent periods of poor diabetic control. In general, sexual function is restored once metabolic control has improved.

The second type of sexual problem is characteristic of diabetes and is often termed 'diabetic impotence'. It has long been thought to exemplify an organically-determined disturbance of sexual function. This is because its most common presentation is with a progressive and irreversible decline in sexual function which occurs when the diabetes is apparently well controlled and the patient is under no identifiable psychological stress. There have

Clinics in Endocrinology and Metabolism — Vol. 11, No. 3, November 1982.

749
0300-595X/82/11.03/749 $03.00 © W. B. Saunders Company Ltd.

been few systematic studies of its clinical features, perhaps because sexual history-taking is a skill which has been relatively ignored in medical training. Recent studies in which sexual function has been comprehensively assessed suggest that the disorder is more varied and extensive than is implied by the term 'diabetic impotence'. For this reason consideration will be given to the effects of diabetes on four distinct aspects of male sexual function.

Erectile function

Difficulty in obtaining or maintaining an erection is undoubtedly the most prominent sexual problem in diabetes. The first recorded case was that of a 30-year-old Glaswegian porter whose problems were summarized in John Rollo's book (1798) as follows: 'He is the father of several children, but since he has been seized with Diabetes — Coitus nullus. Erigitum nunquam: ne quidem semel rigescit.' Several other authors in the pre-insulin era commented on the frequency of the problem. For example, Naunyn (1906) regarded impotence as one of the commonest symptoms, reporting its occurrence both in patients debilitated by loss of sugar and in those relatively untroubled by the disease. Following the introduction of insulin in the 1920s little mention was made of impotence for almost 30 years. In 1950 Simpson stated that persistent impotence was not common 'in patients who have always been controlled with a balanced diet and insulin'. However, since then a series of studies have indicated that between one-third and one-half of diabetic men complain of some degree of erectile failure (Table 1). The interpretation of this finding is problematical since none of the studies have included control groups. Usually comparisons have been drawn with Kinsey's figures (Kinsey, Pomeroy and Martin, 1948), but the validity of this comparison may be questioned in view of the differing methods of case identification and the inadequate definition of normal and abnormal sexual function. A second difficulty in interpretation arises from the absence of information on the prevalence of sexual problems among patients with other chronic physical diseases. This point has been highlighted by the modest study of Lester, Grant and Woodroffe (1980) in which diabetic and non-diabetic outpatients attending follow-up clinics were given a simple questionnaire concerning sexual function. It was found that the incidence of erectile failure was similar in the two populations. This important finding has yet to be replicated.

Table 1. *Prevalence studies of diabetic impotence*

	Number in sample	Age range	Percentage impotent
Rubin and Babbott (1958)	198	16 — 92	55
Schöffling (1960)	314	16 — 65	51
Montenero and Donatone (1962)	436	20 — 65	37
Ellenberg (1971)	200	Not recorded	59
Faerman et al (1972)	299	18 — 50	40
Kolodny et al (1974)	175	18 — 81	49
McCulloch et al (1980)	541	20 — 59	35

The prevalence studies indicate that the number of patients who admit to erectile difficulties increases with age. McCulloch et al (1980) found a prevalence of 5.7 per cent in men aged 20 to 24 years and this rose to 52.4 per cent in men aged 55 to 59 years. It was, thought that like most diabetic complications the frequency of erectile failure was directly related to the duration of the disorder (Schöffling, Federlin and Ditchunheit, 1963), but other studies have either failed to confirm this (Ellenberg, 1971; Kolodny et al, 1974), or they have attributed the relationship to the influence of other factors of probable aetiological importance such as diabetic microangiopathy and neuropathy (McCulloch et al, 1980). In all the studies erectile failure was found to be more common among patients with evidence of neuropathy. It has been suggested that the development of erectile failure is unrelated to the quality of diabetic control (Martin, 1953; Ellenberg, 1971; Kolodny et al, 1974). However, all these studies have relied on the retrospective assessment of metabolic control, a procedure of limited validity. Indirect evidence in support of a relationship between diabetic control and erectile failure comes from the study of McCulloch et al (1980) in which a strong relationship was found between the prevalence of erectile failure and the presence and severity of retinopathy, a complication that may reflect poor metabolic control (Tchobroutsky, 1978).

Most descriptions of the erectile problems of diabetic men have implied there is a uniform clinical picture characterized by a gradual but progressive deterioration in the strength of the patient's erection (for example: Rubin and Babbott, 1958; Cooper, 1972; Kolodny et al, 1974). All erections are said to be affected, including those obtained on waking, on masturbating, and those developed spontaneously through the day. This picture is contrasted with that of 'psychogenic impotence' in which the erectile failure develops rapidly and is confined to certain circumstances. A small study by Kockott et al (1980) suggests that this distinction is valid. Using a semi-structured interview these authors found a clear difference in symptom profile. The ten diabetic patients had a 'prevailing' failure of erection which affected all erections, whereas the erectile problems of the 16 cases of psychogenic impotence were 'situational': their erectile failure was especially prominent during sexual contact with the partner, and under these circumstances the erection was often strong during foreplay, but it tended to decline in strength once vaginal penetration was attempted.

A recent study suggests that the clinical picture of diabetic impotence is more varied than earlier research implied. In this study a detailed sexual history was taken in a standardized fashion from 27 diabetic men with erectile failure (Fairburn et al, 1982). It was found that while difficulty in obtaining or maintaining an erection was usually the first sign of erectile dysfunction, other modes of onset occurred, including late onset premature ejaculation and a heightened ability to obtain an erection. Initially the severity of erectile failure varied from day to day, but this variability progressively declined. Somewhat unexpectedly, it was found that full morning erections were experienced by over half the patients and spontaneous erections by almost one third. Two patients described an alteration in the shape of their erect penis; neither of these patients gave a history of penile trauma, nor was there clinical evidence of Peyronie's disease. It is possible that the change in erectile shape was the result of microvascular abnormalities in the corpora cavernosa.

Ejaculation

Ejaculatory disturbance also occurs in diabetes. The best described disorder is retrograde ejaculation in which semen passes backwards into the bladder rather than forwards along the anterior urethra (Greene, Kelalis and Weeks, 1963; Ellenberg and Weber, 1966; Greene and Kelalis, 1968). This results in the subject experiencing the pumping sensation associated with ejaculation without semen emerging from his penis. Urine passed immediately after ejaculation tends to be cloudy and the diagnosis is confirmed by finding numerous spermatozoa in a post-orgasmic urine specimen. The same clinical phenomenon is a well established complication of bladder neck surgery, bilateral lumbar sympathectomy, and the taking of adrenergic blocking drugs such as guanethidine and phenoxybenzamine. In all these instances, the competence of the internal sphincter of the bladder is thought to be compromised, either physically or pharmacologically, with the result that it fails to close during the propulsive phase of ejaculation.

Other forms of ejaculatory disturbance are also encountered. For example, in some patients who complain of reduced or absent ejaculation, no spermatozoa can be found in postorgasmic urine specimens (Klebanow and MacLeod, 1960). In these cases there may be a genuine decline in semen production, or alternatively interference with its passage into the urethra. In the series of Fairburn et al (1982) over a third of the sample described an absence of the pumping sensation that normally accompanies ejaculation: these patients described semen seeping from their erect or flaccid penis either at or prior to orgasm. This phenomenon did not resemble the emission experienced by those with severe premature ejaculation since it often occurred prior to orgasm. It is also unlikely to have been due to profuse secretion from the periurethral glands since all the patients said it was a novel phenomenon. Instead, it is likely to have been the result of a subtle disruption of the ejaculatory process.

There have been no attempts to study the prevalence of ejaculatory disturbance in diabetes. Retrograde ejaculation is usually cited as the most common disorder, yet in the series of Kolodny et al (1974) only two patients out of 175 diabetic men had retrograde ejaculation whereas 85 were impotent. The findings of Fairburn et al (1982) suggests that these problems may be underreported since almost half their patients had some form of ejaculatory disorder.

Spermatogenesis

Despite the early claims that testicular atrophy and infertility are common in untreated or poorly controlled diabetic men (cf. Rodriguez-Rigau, 1980), more recent studies have found that fertility and sperm density are not affected in patients with well controlled diabetes or mild carbohydrate intolerance (Klebenow and MacLeod, 1960; Bartak, Josifko and Horakova, 1975; Spellacy et al, 1979; Paz et al, 1977). The effects of diabetes on sperm motility is disputed (Hicks, Rojas and Rosado, 1973; Paz et al, 1977). Spermatogenic infertility is not common in male diabetics, but among those with retrograde ejaculation ejaculatory infertility may occur.

Sexual appetite

In most descriptions of diabetic impotence sexual appetite is said to remain intact despite the profound impairment of erectile function (Rubin and Babbott, 1958; Cooper, 1972; Kolodny et al, 1974). However, two recent studies have found a reduction in sexual appetite in over a quarter of their samples (Jensen et al, 1979; McCulloch et al, 1980). One explanation for this apparent contradiction may lie in changes in sexual appetite over time. Fairburn et al (1982) found that most sexual difficulties arose in the context of an intact appetite for sex, but in almost half their cases this subsequently declined. These authors thought that the decline reflected a secondary psychological reaction to sexual 'failure'. Sexual appetite may of course be impaired in the absence of erectile dysfunction; however, there is no evidence to suggest that this occurs any more commonly among diabetics than non-diabetics.

In conclusion, it appears that the sexual problems of diabetic men are more varied and complex than the traditional concept of diabetic impotence implies. Erectile failure is the most common problem, but ejaculatory changes and disturbed sexual appetite also occur, either in unison or independently of one another. The natural history of these disturbances is largely unknown, although the clinical impression is that they are progressive and irreversible.

AETIOLOGY

Our understanding of the aetiology of these sexual problems is hampered by ignorance over the psychophysiological mechanisms underlying the normal male sexual response. However, it is well recognized that sexual function is a complex psychosomatic phenomenon in which physical and psychological processes interact.

Physical Factors

Endocrine

Whether hormonal abnormalities are of relevance to the sexual problems of diabetic men is uncertain. Some endocrine abnormalities have been detected, but their significance is questionable. Rather than contributing to the sexual problem, they may be secondary changes, or a consequence of diabetes itself.

Clinical reports in the pre-insulin era suggested that erectile failure and testicular atrophy were common among untreated male diabetics. Animal studies found a reduction in androgen production, Leydig cell numbers and LH receptors which was proportional to the duration and severity of hyperglycaemia and reversible with insulin administration (Hunt and Bailey, 1961; Foglia et al, 1969; Charreau et al, 1978; Paz et al, 1978). These findings led to the suggestion that insulin deficiency was the primary cause of 'diabetic impotence'. However, it has since become apparent that the introduction of insulin has had no effect on the association between diabetes and erectile dysfunction.

In 1963 Schöffling and colleagues found that patients with diabetic impotence had a reduced population of Leydig cells and diminished urinary excretion of testosterone metabolites. However, subsequent research utilizing radioimmunoassays of plasma hormones has found no difference in mean plasma testosterone concentrations between impotent diabetics, potent diabetics and normal controls (Kent, 1966; Ellenberg, 1971; Faerman et al, 1972; Kolodny et al, 1974; Wright et al, 1976; Jensen et al, 1979). This observation complements the work of Faerman et al (1972) who found no abnormalities in Leydig cell number and morphology in the testicular biopsies of seven impotent diabetic men. Furthermore, they found no differences in the in vitro testicular metabolism of ^{3}H-pregnenolone between impotent diabetic patients and control subjects with varicocoeles.

Recent studies have suggested that the picture is more complicated than previously envisaged. Geisthovel et al (1975) found that impotent diabetic men have a significantly lower free plasma testosterone and an impaired HCG response compared with potent diabetic controls, and Daubresser et al (1978) found diminished total plasma testosterone in both diabetic and non-diabetic impotent men compared with potent controls. On the basis of these findings, it was suggested that the Leydig cell dysfunction might reflect the low coital frequency of impotent subjects. However, subsequent research has found lower plasma total and free testosterone levels in diabetic men as compared with normal control, irrespective of whether or not there were sexual problems (Shahwan, Spathis and Fry, 1978; Ando et al, 1979; Gattucio et al, 1979). This suggests that Leydig cell dysfunction in diabetics may be secondary to the duration and severity of metabolic disturbance and its treatment, and its association with disturbed sexual function might simply be coincidental. These findings, together with the apparent ineffectiveness of androgen replacement, have led to the conclusion that androgen deficiency is of little relevance to the sexual problems of male diabetics.

Studies of the hypothalamic-pituitary function of diabetic men have been no less confusing. Again Schöffling's group provided the initial impetus by demonstrating low total urinary gonadotrophic activity in some impotent diabetic men (Schöffling, Federlin and Ditschunheit, 1963). The majority of subsequent studies employing radioimmunoassay have found normal basal plasma gonadotrophin levels and normal response to GnRH stimulation among both impotent and potent diabetic men (Rastogi, Chakraborti and Sinha, 1974; Daubresser et al, 1978; Gattucio et al, 1979; Jensen et al, 1979). However, some workers have found that diabetic men have an impaired LH response to GnRH stimulation despite normal basal gonadotrophin levels (Distiller et al, 1975; Wright et al, 1976; Shahwan et al, 1978), and Ando et al (1979) found that young diabetic men with good glycaemic control had high basal LH levels and a prolonged response to GnRH stimulation. Our own studies have found that diabetic men have normal total plasma testosterone levels but significantly increased SHBG-binding capacity (Wu and colleagues, 1981 unpublished observations). This implies that the unbound and biologically active fraction of testosterone is reduced. Basal LH concentration and response to GnRH stimulation, however, are not significantly different from those of normal age-matched controls. These results suggest that the pituitary gonadotrophin production of diabetic men is impaired or inappropriately 'normal' in the presence of low free testosterone. Furthermore, it is important to note that we found no significant differences in any of these hormonal parameters between the impotent and potent diabetic subjects. The prolactin levels were normal in all those diabetic men who had intact renal function and who were not taking psychotropic drugs; this finding is in agreement with those of several other recent studies (Shahwan, Spathis and Fry, 1978; Jensen et al, 1979; Lester, Woodroffe and Smith, 1981).

At present it is difficult to evaluate the relevance of hormonal factors to the sexual problems of diabetic men. Our findings are in keeping with the overall impression that the hormonal abnormalities that have been demonstrated may not be of primary aetiological importance since similar changes are encountered among potent diabetic controls. However, it must be emphasized that the relationship between individual aspects of the male sexual response (erection, ejaculation and sexual appetite) and endocrine function has yet to be explored. Furthermore, there has been a failure to take account of variables such as the quality of metabolic control, the subjects' age and treatment, and the circadian and circhoral variations in testosterone and gonadotrophin levels. For these reasons further research is required.

Vascular

An adequate arterial blood supply is a prerequisite for the development and maintenance of a full erection. Large vessel disease may result in erectile failure, as in the Leriche syndrome, and it is possible that small vessel disease may also contribute to erectile dysfunction (Ginestie and Romieu, 1978). For example, Herman, Adar and Rubinstein (1978) found significantly greater stenosis in the internal pudendal arteries of impotent patients as compared with potent controls. (The role of vascular factors in the aetiology of erectile failure is discussed in detail in Chapters 7 and 8.)

There is conflicting evidence regarding the significance of structural vascular disease to the erectile problems of diabetic men. One angiographic study found an impaired blood supply to the corpora cavernosa (Fournier and Huguet, 1968), but this observation remains unconfirmed. Penile blood pressure studies suggest that the blood supply to the penis may be impaired in some diabetic patients (Gaskell, 1971; Abelson, 1975; Engel, Burnham and Carter, 1978; Karacan et al, 1978; Karacan, 1980), but these findings require cautious interpretation in view of the paucity of normative data, and the poor correlation between penile blood pressure and the results of angiography (Engel, Burnham and Carter, 1978).

It is possible that instead of there being a structural vascular lesion, there might be a disturbance in the vascular changes responsible for erection formation and maintenance. Both arterial inflow and venous drainage might be disrupted, and if this were the case it is likely that it would be secondary to autonomic nerve damage. Recent technical advances in the study of the psychophysiology of the male sexual response may clarify this issue, as may radioisotope techniques for investigating penile blood flow (Shirai, Nakamura and Matsuda, 1973; Shirai and Nakamura, 1975).

Neurological

Erectile failure in diabetes is widely regarded as a symptom of autonomic nerve damage. This is based upon the clinical and epidemiological association between symptoms of autonomic neuropathy and disturbed erectile function (Clarke, Ewing and Campbell, 1979). However, the absence of satisfactory tests of erectile function have precluded the demonstration of a definite causal relationship between autonomic nerve dysfunction and erectile failure. Strong indirect evidence comes from investigation into the relationship between bladder dysfunction and impotence since the bladder and penis share the same peripheral autonomic pathways. In the best-known study of this type, Ellenberg (1971) found abnormal cystometrograms in 37 out of 45 impotent diabetic patients compared with three out of 30 potent diabetic controls. Buck et al (1976) have since reported similar findings. Further indirect evidence comes from the observation that the bulbocavernosus reflex response latency is prolonged in impotent diabetic men compared with potent, non-diabetic controls (Karacan, 1980); no data on potent diabetic men were provided.

More direct support for the role of autonomic nerve damage comes from the work of Faerman ct al (1974). They performed histochemical studies on the corpora cavernosa of five impotent diabetic men and five impotent nondiabetic controls. Four of the five impotent diabetics had evidence of autonomic nerve abnormalities, whereas no abnormalities were present in the control group. In two similar studies, Melman and Henry (1979) and Melman et al (1980) found lower noradrenaline concentrations in the erectile tissue of impotent diabetic men compared with a mixed group of non-diabetic controls; again there were no comparison figures for potent diabetic men.

Overall, there is compelling evidence to suggest that pelvic autonomic neuropathy contributes to the erectile problems of many diabetic men. However, it is important to note that erectile failure is significantly more common than the other features of autonomic neuropathy. There are many patients who present with erectile dysfunction as an isolated feature and who have normal cardiovascular reflexes. When these men are followed prospectively a substantial number develop symptoms of more widespread autonomic neuropathy and, in addition, abnormalities on autonomic nerve function tests (Ewing, Campbell and Clark, 1980). In the autonomic nerve supply to the cardiovascular system it has been found that parasympathetic fibres are damaged before the sympathetic nerves (Ewing, Campbell and Clark, 1981). It is possible that the long parasympathetic fibres to the pelvic organs are the most vulnerable of all the autonomic nerves. This would explain why erectile failure may be the earliest and most common feature of diabetic autonomic neuropathy.

Other physical factors

Sexual function is sensitive to many influences in addition to the endocrine, vascular and neurological factors discussed earlier. These include other physical diseases, acute and chronic alcohol abuse, and the ingestion of any of a wide variety of drugs (Furlow, 1979a; Kolodny, Masters and Johnson, 1979). Fairburn et al (1982) found that in over a third of their diabetic patients with erectile failure physical factors of this type might have contributed to the sexual problem.

Psychological Factors

It is widely accepted that psychological factors are of prime importance in the aetiology of most sexual problems. However, the possible role of such factors in the origin and maintenance of the sexual problems of diabetic men has received scant attention, a neglect which probably stems from the assumption that these problems are exclusively physical in origin.

There are several ways in which psychological factors might contribute. First, since both diabetes and sexual problems are common, it is to be expected that some cases will arise from the chance association of the two. Under these circumstances the sexual problem is likely to result from similar psychological processes to those operating among non-diabetic men. The psychological factors most commonly implicated are as follows:

1. ignorance and misunderstandings about sex;
2. negative attitudes towards sex;
3. poor self-esteem and self-image;
4. marital disharmony;
5. anxiety over sexual performance.

It is possible that these factors might be unusually prevalent among diabetic men, thereby explaining in part the raised prevalence of sexual dysfunction. For example, there is an impression that depression and poor self-esteem are relatively common among diabetics (Tattersall, 1981). Furthermore, it is self-evident that diabetes poses problems not only for the individual but also for his spouse (Campbell and McCulloch, 1979), and these problems may in turn increase the likelihood of marital conflict. However, there is no reason to suspect that diabetic men are exceptionally ill-informed about sex, unduly negative in their attitudes, or especially prone to performance anxiety.

If these psychological 'risk' factors were contributing, it might be expected that the clinical picture would resemble that associated with psychogenic impotence. This was partly confirmed by Fairburn and colleagues (1982), who found that in the presence of marital disharmony or a history of earlier sexual difficulties (assumed to be indicative of a psychological vulnerability to sexual dysfunction), patients were more likely to have intact morning and spontaneous erections and a reduced appetite for sex.

Whatever the primary 'cause' of a sexual problem, there is invariably a secondary psychological reaction in the individual and his partner. The reaction most characteristic of men with erectile failure is performance anxiety, and, not surprisingly, this tends to worsen matters, thereby establishing a vicious circle. In addition, sexual problems may threaten the individual's self-esteem, and they can lead to marital disharmony. Fairburn and colleagues (1982) were able to distinguish four types of reaction among diabetic men with erectile dysfunction. The most common was anxiety over the decline in sexual performance which was eventually followed by a degree of sexual avoidance together with a reduced appetite for sex. After a variable period some of these patients began to accept the problem; their view was that they should make the most of their limited sexual capabilities. This attitude appeared to develop gradually and its development was facilitated by the realization that such difficulties are prone to occur in diabetes. A minority of patients had this attitude from the outset. Other patients seemed unperturbed by the disturbance in sexual function, stating that sex had never been of great importance to them. The majority of wives reacted sympathetically to their husband's sexual difficulties. In those cases in which there was an adverse reaction the wife tended to blame herself, thinking that she was no longer attractive to her spouse. However, in a few cases the reaction was of anger and resentment, and not surprisingly in these instances there was often a history of marital discord.

ASSESSMENT

The aims of assessment are to obtain an accurate description of the sexual problem, to gauge the relative contributions of both physical and psychological factors, and to plan treatment.

Description of the sexual problem

A description of the sexual problem should be obtained from both the patient and his partner. Information is required on the present state of the problem as well as its onset and development. When taking the history it is important to consider concurrent changes in the patient's physical and psychological state. For example, the problem may have started following the prescription of a drug with adverse effects on sexual function, or it may have begun during a period of marital conflict. Systematic enquiry into present sexual function is essential. It is important to know whether the patient ever obtains erections, and if so, under what circumstances. Disturbances of ejaculation and sexual appetite should also be recorded. The secondary psychological reaction is of great significance: the patient and his partner should be routinely asked about performance anxiety, the avoidance of sex, and secondary effects on self-esteem and the marriage. With tactful but explicit questioning, a clear picture of the problem will usually emerge. Sometimes this will resemble the diabetic or psychogenic stereotypes discussed earlier, but more often the clinical picture will be a mixture of the two (Schiavi and Hogan, 1979; Fairburn et al, 1982).

Physical assessment

Having obtained a description of the problem, the relative contributions of physical and psychological factors must be considered. A systematic medical history and physical examination is always required. With the diabetic patient special emphasis must be placed on symptoms and signs suggestive of the aetiological factors mentioned earlier. The history of pubertal development and previous sexual functioning should be documented in order to establish the normality or otherwise of hypo-thalamic-pituitary-testicular function. The presence of neuropathic symptoms, both autonomic and peripheral, should also be sought. For example, bladder symptoms such as diminished frequency of micturition, increased urinary volume at each micturition, slow urine stream, and retention and overflow may be indicative of disturbances in the sacral autonomic nerve supply to the bladder, and hence also the penis. The presence of peripheral vascular disease, especially with symptoms involving the thighs and buttocks, should raise the possibility of major pelvic vascular occlusions. In addition, patients with diabetes are often taking drugs which may disturb sexual function, the most common being anti-hypertensive agents and psychotropic drugs (Horowitz and Goble, 1979; Kolodny, Masters and Johnson, 1979). Alcohol abuse is a further factor which must be considered.

The physical examination should include an assessment of androgenic status. Body habitus; facial, body and pubic hair; gynaecomastia; testicular size and consistency; and the presence of varicocoeles should be documented. External genitalia should be examined for congenital deformities, plaques associated with Peyronie's disease, and the presence of balanitis or phimosis. The absence or diminution of testicular sensation may indicate damage to the afferent sympathetic supply of the testis (Campbell et al, 1974), whereas the absence of the bulbocavernosus reflex is indicative of lesions in the sacral visceral pathway (S2-4) (Blaivas, Zayed and Labib, 1981). The clinical features of autonomic neuropathy include postural hypotension, resting tachycardia, anhydrosis in the lower limbs, and small and slowly reacting pupils (Clark, Ewing and Campbell, 1979). A glove-and-stocking distribution of sensory loss, followed later by muscle weakness and wasting due to polyneuropathy, may also be found. The peripheral pulses should be examined for evidence of occlusion; however, it must be emphasized that intact lower limb pulses do not necessarily exclude major occlusions of the pelvic arteries.

The presence of visceral autonomic neuropathy can be confirmed by the assessment of cardiovascular reflex abnormalities (Ewing, 1978). However, these tests do not assess the integrity of the pelvic autonomic nerve supply, and erectile failure often occurs in the presence of normal cardiovascular reflexes (Ewing et al, 1973). Of greater relevance therefore are cystometrograms, and urodynamic studies can demonstrate abnormal detrusor activity and loss of bladder sensation secondary to neuropathic involvement of the pelvic autonomic supply (Frimhodt-Møller, 1978; Bradley, 1980). However, these procedures are invasive and normative data are scanty.

Furthermore, despite the common nerve supply to the bladder and the penis, diabetic cystopathy is only variably related to erectile failure (Frimodt-Møller, 1980).

Assessment of the vascular supply to the penis is more straightforward although the techniques are still in their infancy. The measurement of penile blood pressure using a digital cuff and portable ultrasound Doppler system provides a convenient means for detecting local vascular abnormalities (Engel, Burnham and Carter, 1978; Nath et al, 1981), and a similar technique may be used to measure blood flow transcutaneously over the six penile arteries (Jevitch, 1980). If microvascular surgery is contemplated, translumbar angiography can be performed to localize the sites of stenosis (Herman, Adar and Rubinstein, 1978).

The metabolic assessment of diabetic patients with erectile failure should include basal estimations of plasma testosterone, gonadotrophins and prolactin. Single estimations in the morning are sufficient. If the values obtained are borderline or abnormal, they may be supplemented by multiple estimations and dynamic testing of the pituitary and testicular reserves. It is also important to assess liver and renal function by measuring serum plasma transaminases, alkaline phosphatase, creatinine, and electrolytes. The quality of glycaemic control can be roughly assessed by urinanalysis or the measurement of plasma glucose; a more accurate assessment may be obtained using glycosylated haemoglobin, a test which measures diabetic control over the previous month (Citrin, Elws and Skyler, 1980).

The introduction of surgical techniques for the treatment of irreversible erectile failure has highlighted the need for direct means of assessing the integrity of the erectile response. Two approaches are being developed. The first is the measurement of psychophysiological responses to erotic stimuli. This is a highly specialized technique which has only recently been applied to clinical populations. The second is the study of nocturnal erections. This procedure is simpler, but there are many difficulties inherent in the interpretation of its findings (see Chapter 10).

Psychological assessment

The assessment of the contribution of psychological factors should focus on the five major areas discussed earlier. These can be explored in one or two interviews with the patient and his partner.

Ignorance and misunderstanding about sex. Many patients and their partners have unrealistic expectations regarding the effects of diabetes on sexual function. Often these are not voiced and sometimes they are not shared. For example, the diabetic man who is anticipating erectile problems may assume that once a degree of erectile failure develops his sex life is over, whereas his partner may wish to continue love-making, accepting that this may have to change in style.

Negative attitudes towards sex. The ejaculatory changes experienced by some diabetic men may be distasteful to them, or more often their partner. This is particularly common in those cases in which semen seeps out of the penis as soon as the patient is even moderately aroused. If one or both partners find this unpleasant, love-making may be abandoned despite sexual function being relatively intact. In some cases it emerges that sex had always been viewed as 'messy' or 'dirty'.

Poor self-esteem and self-image. Depression from any cause tends to be associated with a reduction in sexual appetite. Many diabetic patients live in the fear of physical complications. While knowledge that erectile failure is associated with diabetes can be reassuring in the sense that it absolves the patient from 'responsibility' for the problem, it has sinister connotations since erectile failure then becomes a harbinger of further long-term complications. An evaluation of the patient's mood and self-esteem is therefore an important part of assessment.

Marital disharmony. Conflict and resentment, especially when complicated by poor communication, often results in sexual difficulties. As mentioned earlier, there is no doubt that diabetes and its associated disabilities creates problems for both partners. For example, increasing disability can lead to inevitable, but nevertheless resented, shifts in role. Even in marriages in which communication is good there can be difficulties adjusting to such changes, and in marriages where problems already exist, conflict may erupt with secondary repercussions on the sexual relationship. In order to assess the quality of the relationship it is essential to interview the sexual partner who, in the majority of cases, will be more than willing to cooperate.

Anxiety over sexual performance. Patients often view a deterioration in their sexual function as a 'failure' on their part. As a result they become morbidly self-conscious during love-making and profoundly anxious over the quality of their sexual performance. This performance anxiety has a notoriously deleterious effect on sexual function and it may lead to the total avoidance of sex. It can be detected by simple direct questioning.

MANAGEMENT

The aim of management is to help the patient and his partner enjoy sexual function to the full within whatever limits are set by irreversible factors. The first task is therefore to correct any reversible physical factors which might be contributing to the sexual problem. Improving the quality of metabolic control may help those patients with the non-specific type of sexual problem that is associated with many debilitating disorders, but it does not appear to influence the progressive decline in erectile function often found in diabetes. Nevertheless, improving the patient's general state of health can sometimes be beneficial. Whenever possible, it is worth exploring the effect of discontinuing any drugs which have adverse effects on sexual function; but this is not always possible since the control of blood pressure and certain other symptoms must take precedence. Finally, if excessive alcohol consumption is a problem this should receive treatment in its own right.

The second task is to tackle those psychological factors which appear to be contributing to the sexual disorder. Although primary psychological problems do not appear to be especially common, there is almost invariably a secondary psychological reaction and, as mentioned earlier, this tends to worsen the already curtailed sexual performance.

The importance of providing information and advice cannot be over-stated. Most patients want to know the likely contribution of irreversible physical factors. While it has been suggested that providing information of this type encourages the patient to adopt a fatalistic attitude to the problem (Renshaw, 1976, 1978), this is unlikely if the patient and his partner are given positive advice on how to approach their sexual problem. This advice usually incorporates the 'prescription' of non-coital sexual exercises known to diminish performance anxiety (Fairburn, Dickerson and Greenwood, 1982): for some patients with severe erectile failure of physical origin, these exercises may be the only form of sexual activity available to them. In addition, these patients need advice on how to adapt to irreversible changes in sexual function: for example, by using alternative positions for sexual intercourse, or exploring novel methods of stimulation such as oro-genital contact. Such advice must be tailored to suit each couple: proposing that they engage in practices which they regard as perverse is clearly counter-productive.

It is important to be alert to more widespread difficulties within the relationship, as well as problems such as depression and low self-esteem. Often by openly discussing these problems with the couple a new perspective can be thrown upon them. The partner can be most helpful: for example, by demonstrating her continuing affection for him despite his diabetes, by indicating that she is still attracted to him, and by explaining that it is their relationship which is important. Should the clinician be uncertain on how best to manage the psychological components of the problem, help may be sought from a local sexual problems clinic or liaison psychiatrist. There is undoubtedly a strong case for one or more members of the diabetic clinic team (medical or non-medical) to be experienced in sex therapy, and in particular in the management of the sexual problems of the disabled. Systematic research into the management of these sexual problems is required.

Finally, mention should be made of surgical approaches to the treatment of erectile failure. If arterial insufficiency appears to be the major cause of erectile dysfunction, Michal et al (1977) have advocated corporal revascularization by small artery grafting (see Chapter 8). The integrity of the corpora cavernosa must be assessed beforehand by a cavernosogram (Fitzpatrick and Cooper, 1975) in order to exclude conditions such as Peyronie's disease which might preclude the restoration of potency. Experience with this type of operation is at present limited and the results are largely unfavourable (Scott, 1980).

Over the past 15 years, however, successful operations have been devised to implant synthetic penile prostheses into the corpora cavernosa. The prostheses are of two main types: the semi-rigid Small-Carrion silicone implant (Small, 1976), and the Scott-Bradley inflatable prosthesis (Furlow,

1979b; Scott et al, 1979). The complication rates in most centres are fairly low, and by using prophylactic antibiotics and carefully selecting appropriately-sized implants the incidence of infection and extrusion is no higher among diabetic patients (Chaikin, Carion and Politano, 1981). The surgical success rates with the two types of prosthesis are similar and each has its own advantages and draw-backs (Malloy, Wein and Carpincello, 1980). However, it must be noted that while these procedures provide the patient with a stiff penis, its resemblance to a natural erection is limited.

The long-term outcome of penile prosthetic surgery has yet to be studied. Note has been taken of the surgical outcome, but the psychosexual effects of these operations has been relatively ignored. Sotile (1979) has argued that the stability of the patient's relationship with his sexual partner should be assessed preoperatively, and that care should be taken to ensure that both have realistic expectations regarding the effects of implantation. The factors that may be associated with a favourable outcome include a stable marital relationship, normal premorbid sexual function, intact sexual appetite and unimpaired genital sensation and orgasmic capacity (Schiavi, 1980).

Requests for penile surgery should be treated with caution. Seagreaves et al (1981) have reported that it is not unusual for men to request penile surgery because they are impotent with their wives while being sexually potent with their mistresses! Before referral to a surgeon is contemplated, it would seem judicious to explore the benefits of less drastic forms of management.

Ejaculatory infertility may be a problem in diabetic men with retrograde ejaculation. Many different methods have been used to recover sperm from the bladder with the minimum contamination by urine, the osmolality and pH of which can be raised by fluid restriction and the administration of alkali (Glazerman et al, 1976). The recovered sperm can then be used for artificial insemination, with or without prior washing procedures. An alternative approach is to encourage anterograde ejaculation, either pharmacologically using alpha-adrenergic stimulants, or mechanically with a full bladder (Stockamp, Schreiter and Altwein, 1974; Crich and Jequier, 1978). None of these approaches has a high success rate.

SUMMARY

Diabetic men are prone to a variety of sexual problems. It is probable that most of these sexual difficulties are the result of a progressive physical disorder upon which a psychological reaction is superimposed. Assessment needs to take account of both the physical and psychological components of the problem. The aim of management is to help the patient and his partner enjoy sexual function to the full within whatever limits are set by irreversible factors. Management therefore involves correcting potentially reversible physical and psychological factors, and helping the patient and his partner adapt to the remaining irreversible changes in sexual function. Using this approach it may be possible to improve the prognosis of what in the past has been dismissed as an intractable clinical problem.

REFERENCES

Abelson, D. (1975) Diagnostic value of the penile pulse and blood pressure: a Doppler study of impotence in diabetics. *Journal of Urology,* **113,** 636-639.

Andó, S., Rubens, R., Polosa, P. & Vermeulen, A. (1979) Hypothalamic-pituitary-gonadal function in male diabetics. In *Recent Progress in Andrology* (Ed.) Fabbrini, A. & Steinberger, E. pp. 359-366. New York: Academic Press.

Bartak, V., Josifko, M. & Horakova, M. (1975) Juvenile diabetes and human sperm quality. *International Journal of Fertility,* **20,** 30-32.

Blaivas, J. G., Zayed, A. A. H. & Labib, K. B. (1981) The bulbocavernosus reflex in urology: a prospective study of 299 patients. *Journal of Urology,* **126,** 179-199.

Bradley, W. E. (1980) Diagnosis of urinary bladder dysfunction in diabetes mellitus. *Annals of Internal Medicine,* **92** (Part 2), 323-326.

Buck, A. C., Reed, P. I., Siddiq, Y. K., Chisholm, G. D. & Fraser, T. R. (1976) Bladder dysfunction and neuropathy in diabetics. *Diabetologia,* **12,** 251-258.

Campbell, I. W. & McCulloch, D. K. (1979) Marital problems in diabetics. *Practitioner,* **223,** 343-347.

Campbell, I. W., Ewing, D. J., Clarke, B. F. & Duncan, L. J. P. (1974) Testicular pain sensation in diabetic autonomic neuropathy. *British Medical Journal,* **ii,** 638-639.

Chaikin, H., Carion, H. & Politano, V. (1981) Complications of the Small-Carrion penile prosthesis: long-term follow-up. *Journal of Urology,* **126,** 44-45.

Charreau, H. E., Calvo, J. C., Tesone, M., de Souz Valle, L. B. & Barono, J. L. (1978) Insulin regulation of Leydig cell luteinizing hormone receptors. *Journal of Biological Chemistry,* **253,** 2504-2506.

Citrin, W., Elws, G. J. & Skyler, J. S. (1980) Glycosylated hemoglobin: a tool in identifying psychological problems. *Diabetes Care,* **3,** 563-564.

Clarke, B. F., Ewing, D. J. & Campbell, I. W. (1979) Diabetic autonomic neuropathy. *Diabetologia,* **17,** 195-212.

Cooper, A. J. (1972) Diagnosis and management of 'endocrine impotence'. *British Medical Journal,* **ii,** 34-36.

Crich, J. P. & Jequier, A. M. (1978) Infertility in men with retrograde ejaculation: the action of urine on sperm motility, and a simple method for achieving anterograde ejaculation. *Fertility and Sterility,* **30,** 572-576.

Daubresser, J-C., Meuenier, J-C., Wilmotte, J. & Luyckx, A. S. (1978) Pituitary-testicular axis in diabetic men with and without sexual impotence. *Diabetes and Metabolism* (Paris), **4,** 233-237.

Distiller, L. A., Sagel, J., Morley, J. E., Joffe, B. F. & Seftel, H. C. (1975) Pituitary responsiveness to luteinizing hormone releasing hormone in insulin-dependent diabetes mellitus. *Diabetes,* **24,** 378-380.

Ellenberg, M. (1971) Impotence in diabetes: the neurologic factor. *Annals of Internal Medicine,* **75,** 213-219.

Ellenberg, M. & Weber, H. (1966) Retrograde ejaculation in diabetic neuropathy. *Annals of Internal Medicine,* **65,** 1237-1246.

Engel, G., Burnham, S. J. & Carter, M. F. (1978) Penile blood pressure in evaluation of erectile impotence. *Fertility and Sterility,* **30,** 687-690.

Ewing, D. J. (1978) Cardiovascular reflexes and autonomic neuropathy. *Clinical Science and Molecular Medicine,* **55,** 321-327.

Ewing, D. J., Campbell, I. W. & Clarke, B. F. (1980) The natural history of diabetic autonomic neuropathy. *Quarterly Journal of Medicine,* **193,** 95-108.

Ewing, D. J., Campbell, I. W. & Clarke, B. F. (1981) Heart rate changes in diabetes mellitus. *Lancet,* **i,** 183-185.

Ewing, D. J., Campbell, I. W., Burt, A. A. & Clarke, B. F. (1973) Vascular reflexes in diabetic autonomic neuropathy. *Lancet,* **ii,** 1354-1356.

Faerman, I., Vilar, O., Rivarola, M. A., Rosner, J. M., Jadzinsky, M. N., Fox, D., Perez Loret, A., Bernstein-Hahn, L. & Saraceni, D. (1972) Impotence and diabetes. Studies of androgenic function in diabetic impotent males. *Diabetes,* **21,** 23-30.

Faerman, I., Blocer, I., Fox, D., Jadzinsky, M. N. & Rapaport, M. (1974) Impotence and diabetes. Histological studies of the autonomic nervous fibres of the corpora cavernosa in impotent diabetic males. *Diabetes,* **23,** 971-976.

Fairburn, C. G., Dickerson, M. G. & Greenwood, J. (1982) *Sexual Problems and their Management.* Edinburgh: Churchill Livingstone (in press).

Fairburn, C. G., Wu, F. C. W., McCulloch, D. K., Borsay, D. Q., Ewing, D. J., Clarke, B. F. & Bancroft, J. H. J. (1982) The clinical features of diabetic impotence: a preliminary study. *British Journal of Psychiatry,* **140,** 447-452.

Fitzpatrick, P. J. & Cooper, J. F. (1975) A cavernogram study of the valvular competence of the human deep dorsal vein. *Journal of Urology,* **113,** 497-499.

Foglia, V. G., Rosner, J. M., Cattaneo de Peralta, Raymos, M. & Lema, B. E. (1969) Sexual disturbances in the male diabetic rat. *Hormone and Metabolic Research,* **1,** 72-77.

Fournier, A. M. & Huguet, J. F. (1968) Vascularization du bulbe caverneux. Aspect normal et pathologique. (cas particulier du diabète). *Journal de Radiologie, d'électrologie et de Médecine Nucleaire,* **49,** 515-517.

Frimodt-Møller, C. (1978) Diabetic cystopathy: a review of the urodynamic and clinical features of neurogenic bladder dysfunction in diabetes mellitus. *Danish Medical Bulletin,* **25,** 49-60.

Frimodt-Møller, C. (1980) Diabetic cystopathy: epidemiology and related disorders. *Annals of Internal Medicine,* **92** (Part 2), 318-321.

Furlow, W. L. (1979a) Diagnosis and treatment of male erectile failure. *Diabetes Care,* **2,** 18-25.

Furlow, W. L. (1979b) Inflatable penile prosthesis: Mayo Clinic experience with 175 patients. *Urology,* **13,** 166-171.

Gaskell, P. (1971) The importance of penile blood pressure in cases of impotence. *Canadian Medical Association Journal,* **105,** 1047-1051.

Gattucio, F., Porcelli, P., Morici, V., Lo Bartolo, G. & Janni, A. (1979) The hypothalamic-pituitary-testicular axis in diabetic subjects. In *Recent Progress in Andrology* (ed.) Fabbrini, A. & Steinberger, E. 351-358. New York: Academic Press.

Geisthovel, W., Niedergerke, U., Morgner, K. D., Willms, B. & Mitzkat, H. J. (1975) Androgustatus bei mannlichen Diabetikern. *Medizinishe Klinik,* **70,** 1417-1423.

Ginestie, J-F. & Romieu, A. (1978) *Radiologic Exploration of Impotence.* Martinus Nijkoff Medical Division, London.

Glazerman, M., Lunenfeld, B., Potashnik, G., Oelsner, G. & Beer, R. (1976) Retrograde ejaculation: pathophysiological aspects and report of two successfully treated cases. *Fertility and Sterility,* **27,** 796-800.

Greene, L. F. & Kelalis, P. P. (1968) Retrograde ejaculation of semen due to diabetic neuropathy. *Journal of Urology,* **98,** 693-696.

Greene, L. F., Kelalis, P. P. & Weeks, R. E. (1963) Retrograde ejaculation of semen due to diabetic neuropathy. *Fertility and Sterility,* **14,** 617-625.

Herman, A., Adar, R. & Rubinstein, Z. (1978) Vascular lesions associated with impotence in diabetic and non-diabetic arterial occlusive disease. *Diabetes,* **27,** 975-981.

Hicks, J. J., Rojas, L. & Rosado, A. (1973) Insulin regulation of spermatozoa metabolism. *Endocrinology,* **92,** 833-839.

Horowitz, J. D. & Goble, A. J. (1979) Drugs and impaired male sexual function. *Drugs,* **18,** 206-217.

Hunt, E. L. & Bailey, D. W. (1961) The effect of alloxan diabetes on the reproductive system of young male rats. *Acta Endocrinologica,* **38,** 432-440.

Jensen, S. B., Hagen, C., Frøland, A. & Petersen, P. B. (1979) Sexual function and pituitary axis in insulin treated diabetic men. *Acta Medica Scandinavica Supplementum,* **624,** 65-68.

Jevitch, M. J. (1980) Importance of penile arterial pulse sound examination in impotence. *Journal of Urology,* **124,** 820-824.

Karacan, I. (1980) Diagnosis of erectile impotence in diabetes mellitus: an objective and specific method. *Annals of Internal Medicine,* **92** (Part 2), 334-337.

Karacan, I., Ware, J. C., Dervent, B., Altinel, A., Thornby, J. I., Williams, R. L., Kaya, N. & Scott, F. B. (1978) Impotence and blood pressure in the flaccid penis: relationship to nocturnal penile tumescence. *Sleep.* **1,** 125-132.

Kent, J. R. (1966) Gonadal function in impotent diabetic males. *Diabetes,* **15,** 537.

Kinsey, A. C., Pomeroy, W. B. & Martin, C. E. (1948) *Sexual Behavior in the Human Male.* Philadelphia: W. B. Saunders.

Klebanow, D. & MacLeod, J. (1960) Semen quality and certain disturbances of reproduction in diabetic men. *Fertility and Sterility,* **11,** 255-261.

Kockott, G., Feil, W., Revenstorf, D., Aldenhoff, J. & Besinger, U. (1980) Symptomatology and psychological aspects of male sexual inadequacy: results of an experimental study. *Archives of Sexual Behavior,* **9,** 457-475.

Kolodny, R. C., Masters, W. H. & Johnson, V. E. (1979) *Textbook of Sexual Medicine.* Boston: Little, Brown.

Kolodny, R. C., Kahn, C. B., Goldstein, H. H. & Barnett, D. M. (1974) Sexual dysfunction in men. *Diabetes,* **23,** 306-309.

Lester, E., Grant, A. J. & Woodroffe, F. J. (1980) Impotence in diabetic and non-diabetic out-patients. *British Medical Journal,* **281,** 354-355.

Lester, E., Woodroffe, F. J. & Smith, R. L. (1981) Prolactin and impotence in diabetes mellitus. *Annals of Clinical Biochemistry,* **18,** 6-8.

Malloy, T. R., Wein, A. J. & Carpincello, V. L. (1980) Comparison of the inflatable penile and the Small-Carrion prosthesis in the surgical treatment of erectile impotence. *Journal of Urology,* **123,** 678-679.

Martin, M. M. (1953) Diabetic neuropathy. *Brain,* **76,** 594-624.

McCulloch, D. K., Campbell, I. W., Wu, F. C., Prescott, R. J. & Clarke, B. F. (1980) The prevalence of diabetic impotence. *Diabetologia,* **18,** 279-283.

Melman, A. & Henry, D. (1979) The possible role of catecholamines of the corpora in penile erection. *Journal of Urology,* **121,** 419-421.

Melman, A., Henry, D. P., Felten, D. L. & O'Connor, B. L. (1980) Alteration of the penile corpora in patients with erectile impotence. *Investigative Urology,* **17,** 474-477.

Michal, V., Kramer, R., Pospíckal, J. & Hejhal, L. (1977) Arterial epigastricocavernous anastomosis for the treatment of sexual impotence. *World Journal of Surgery,* **1,** 515-520.

Montenero, P. & Donatone, E. (1962) Diabète et activité sexuelle chez l'homme. *Le Diabète,* **10,** 327-335.

Nath, R. L., Menzoian, J. O., Kaplan, K. H., McMillan, T. N., Siroky, M. B. & Krane, R. J. (1981) The multiple disciplinary approach to vasculogenic impotence. *Surgery,* **89,** 124-133.

Naunyn, B. (1906) *Der Diabetes Mellitus.* Vienna: Alfred Holder.

Paz, G., Homonnai, Z. T., Ayalon, D., Cordova, T. & Kraicer, P. F. (1977) Immuno-reactive insulin in serum and seminal plasma of diabetic and non-diabetic men and its role in the regulation of spermatozoal activity. *Fertility and Sterility,* **28,** 836-840.

Paz, G., Homonnai, Z. T., Drasnin, N., Sofer, A., Kaplan, R. & Kraicer, P. F. (1978) Fertility of the streptozotocin-diabetic male rat. *Andrologia,* **10,** 127-136.

Rastogi, G. K., Chakraborti, J. & Sinha, M. K. (1974) Serum gonadotrophins (LH and FSH) and their response to synthetic LHRH in diabetic men with and without impotence. *Hormone and Metabolic Research,* **6,** 335-336.

Renshaw, D. C. (1976) Impotence in diabetes mellitus. *Comprehensive Therapy,* **2,** 47-50.

Renshaw, D. C. (1978) Impotence in diabetes. In *Handbook of Sex Therapy* (Ed.) LoPiccolo, J. & LoPiccolo, L. pp. 433-440. New York: Plenum Press.

Rodriguez-Rigau, L. J. (1980) Diabetes and male reproductive function. *Journal of Andrology,* **1,** 105-111.

Rollo, J. (1798) An account of two cases of diabetes mellitus: with remarks as they arose during the progress of the care. In *John Rollo's book.* London: C. Dilly.

Rubin, A. & Babbott, D. (1958) Impotence and diabetes mellitus. *Journal of the American Medical Association,* **168,** 498-500.

Schiavi, R. C. (1980) Psychological treatment of erectile disorders in diabetic patients. *Annals of Internal Medicine,* **92** (Part 2), 337-339.

Schiavi, R. C. & Hogan, B. (1979) Sexual problems in diabetes mellitus: psychological aspects. *Diabetes Care,* **2,** 9-17.

Schöffling, K. (1960) *Störungen der Keimdrüsenfunktion bei männlichen Zuckerkranken.* Stuttgart: Enke.

Schöffling, K., Federlin, K. & Ditschunheit, H. (1963) Disorders of sexual function in male diabetics. *Diabetes,* **12,** 519-527.

Scott, F. B. (1980) Surgical treatment of erectile impotence. *Contemporary Surgery,* **16,** 64-90.

Scott, F. B., Byrd, G. J., Karacan, I., Olsson, P., Beulter, L. E. & Attia, S. L. (1979) Erectile impotence treated with an implantable, inflatable prosthesis. *Journal of the American Medical Association,* **241,** 2609-2612.

Seagraves, R. T., Schoenberg, H. W., Zarins, C. K., Camic, P. & Knoff, J. (1981) Characteristics of erectile dysfunction as a function of medical care system entry point. *Psychosomatic Medicine,* **43,** 227-234.

Shahwan, M. M., Spathis, G. S. & Fry, D. E. (1978) Differences in pituitary and testicular function between diabetic patients on insulin and oral anti-diabetic agents. *Diabetologia,* **15,** 13-17.

Shirai, M. & Nakamura, M. (1975) Diagnostic discrimination between organic and functional impotence by radioisotope penogram with 99mTc04. *Tohoku Journal of Experimental Medicine,* **116,** 9-15.

Shirai, M., Nakamura, M. & Matsuda, S. (1973) Differential diagnosis between functional and organic impotence by radioisotope penogram following visual sexual stimulation. *Tohoku Journal of Experimental Medicine,* **111,** 187-195.

Small, M. P. (1976) Small-Carrion penile prosthesis. *Mayo Clinic Proceedings,* **51,** 336-338.

Sotile, W. M. (1979) The penile prosthesis and diabetic impotence: some caveats. *Diabetes Care,* **2,** 26-30.

Spellacy, W. N., Cantor, B., Snydel, F., Buhi, W. C. & Birk, S. A. (1979) Carbohydrate metabolism and the semen profile: glucose, insulin and sperm counts. *Fertility and Sterility,* **32,** 562-565.

Stockamp, K., Schreiter, F. & Altwein, J. E. (1974) Adrenergic drugs in retrograde ejaculation. *Fertility and Sterility,* **25,** 817-820.

Tattersall, R. B. (1981) Psychiatric aspects of diabetes — a physician's view. *British Journal of Psychiatry,* **139,** 485-493.

Tchobroutsky, G. (1978) Relation of diabetic control to development of microvascular complications. *Diabetologia,* **15,** 143-152.

Wright, A. D., London, D. R., Holder, G., Williams, J. W. & Rudd, B. T. (1976) Luteinizing release hormone tests in impotent diabetic males. *Diabetes,* **25,** 975-977.

10

Assessment of Diabetic Impotence: Measurement of Nocturnal Erections

RAUL C. SCHIAVI
CHARLES FISHER

INTRODUCTION

The frequent association of erectile disorders and diabetes mellitus has been well documented (Schiavi and Hogan, 1979). Increasing evidence suggests that neuropathic and vascular mechanisms (Ellenberg, 1971; Abelson, 1975; Buck et al, 1976; Ewing et al, 1976) but not hormonal mechanisms (Faerman et al, 1972; Rastogi, Chakraborti and Sinha, 1974) are pathogenically responsible for diabetic erectile impotence. The neurovascular impairment may develop over several years, however, and the time of onset and extent of erectile problems are frequently influenced by psychosocial factors. Most prevalent among these are the cultural background of the individual, personality characteristics, his previous sexual experience and competency, and the partner's reaction to the sexual difficulty. The co-existence of possible organic and psychological determinants among diabetics frequently creates considerable problems in differential diagnosis. Until recently the distinction between psychogenic and organic forms of impotence was based mainly on clinical evidence derived from the psychosexual history and the existence of medical conditions known to be associated with erectile disorders. During the last few years several non-invasive procedures have been developed for the objective assessment of organic impairment in erectile capacity. Presently, the assessment of nocturnal penile tumescence (NPT) is one of the most frequently used ancillary procedures for differential diagnosis. Although this method provides potentially valuable diagnostic information, it has not yet been adequately validated and is frequently applied uncritically without knowledge of its limitations or awareness of existing methodological problems.

The present chapter will briefly review the literature on NPT in normal and impotent men, with special emphasis on issues relevant to the validity of this approach for differential diagnosis. Preliminary evidence will be presented on a validational study conducted on diabetic patients. Several procedural aspects of importance for the clinical application of the method will then be considered.

Clinics in Endocrinology and Metabolism — Vol. 11, No. 3, November 1982.
0300-595X/82/11.03/769 $03.00 © 1982 W. B. Saunders Company Ltd.

NORMATIVE INFORMATION

Ohlmeyer (Ohlmeyer, Brilmayer and Hüllstrung, 1944), in the German literature of the 1940s, described a recurrent 85-minute cycle of penile tumescence during sleep, with erectile episodes lasting for about 25 minutes. Aserinsky and Kleitman (1955) noted a close correspondence between the frequency and distribution of these episodes and the occurrence of REM sleep. In the middle 1960s Fisher, Gross and Zuch (1964, 1965) and Karacan (1965 unpublished data) were the first to demonstrate experimentally a close temporal relation between erectile activity and over 80 per cent of REM periods in young adult males. Studies conducted since then in the laboratories of Fisher (Fisher, 1966; Kahn and Fisher, 1969), Karacan (Hursch, Karacan and Williams, 1972; Karacan et al, 1972 a and b) and Jovanović (1972) have gathered considerable normative information on the characteristics of nocturnal penile tumescence. NPT is a consistently observed and relatively stable physiological phenomena in normal men from infancy to old age. Changes in various tumescent parameters occur, however, in relation to age (Kahn and Fisher, 1969; Karacan et al, 1975; Karacan et al, 1976). Total tumescent time declines from age 13 when it constitutes 32 per cent of sleep to 20 per cent in the 60 to 69 age range. The number of erectile episodes similarly decrease from a mean of 6.8 per night in adolescence to 3.5 above age 60. In teenagers and young adults more than 90 per cent of all NPT episodes occur at least in part during an REM period and about 90 per cent of all REM periods are associated with tumescence. This relationship gradually declines to about two-thirds by the age of 60 to 69. Total tumescent time and REM time are approximately equal during the pre-teen years. During puberty, at a time when marked changes in secondary sexual characteristics take place, a rather abrupt increase in total tumescent time occurs relative to REM. Following puberty tumescent time gradually decreases, approximating again the duration of REM. The time during which tumescence actually overlaps with REM sleep (simultaneous REM and tumescence) also shows a decline, with a mean of 102 minutes at ages 13 to 15, 72 minutes at ages 30 to 37, and 50 minutes at ages 60 to 69. Of special interest is the mean frequency of maximum erections in various age groups. Based on a definition of maximum erection as a change in penile circumference between 81 and 100 per cent of the greatest circumference recorded for the subject, Karacan et al (1976) have reported a mean of four maximum tumescent episodes in the 13 to 15 age group, three in the 30 to 39 age group, between 2 and 2.4 in ages 40 to 67, and 1.7 in ages 70 to 79.

The degree to which diurnal events or the psychological state of the individual impinge on NPT is not clear. Recency or amount of sexual activity does not seem to influence NPT. Anxiety manifested in dream content or induced by the experimental situation, on the other hand, does appear to inhibit sleep-related erectile activity (Fisher, 1966; Karacan et al, 1966). The functional significance of NPT is presently unknown. There is indirect evidence (Fisher et al, 1965, 1966; Karacan, 1965) to suggest that REM sleep and penile erection are controlled by independent mechanisms which most often coincide temporally but may be disassociated. An important aspect in need of study is the nature of the relation between the neurophysiological and endocrine processes that subserve erotically-induced erections and REM-related NPT.

NPT AND DIFFERENTIAL DIAGNOSIS

Clinical investigations

Jovanović and Tan-eli (1969) compared nocturnal erections in a group of middle-aged healthy males with those in impotent patients prior to and after treatment with a combined preparation of methyl testosterone and psycho-active agents. Mean estimates of frequency, duration and amplitude of erectile episodes were lower in men with erectile problems than in control subjects, and these values reached normal levels following pharmacological treatment. The authors did not describe the clinical characteristics of the sample of impotent men. In a German monograph which appeared in 1972 Jovanović reported the NPT characteristics of several diagnostic groups of impotent men: neurotics, reactive depressives, manic depressives and schizophrenics, among others. Marked NPT impairment was observed in psychogenically impotent neurotics with absence of full erections; the greatest impairment was noted in patients with endogenous depression. Karacan (1970) was the first to suggest that the assessment of NPT could provide a valuable clinical tool for the diagnosis and prognosis of impotence. He reported preliminary observations on a group of diabetic impotent men: patients who showed NPT responded to psychotherapy and dietary changes with restoration of potency, while those with a complete absence of NPT were assumed to suffer from organic impotence and to have poor prognosis. In 1975 Fisher et al and Karacan et al began publishing systematic information on the assessment of NPT in the differential diagnosis of erectile impotence. They proposed the notion that in psychogenic impotence REM erections are normal, in marked discrepancy with patients' daytime performance, while in the organically impotent, nocturnal erections correspond closely to the patient's impaired waking erectile capacity.

Since then several studies have specifically used the NPT method for the assessment of diabetic erectile impotence. Karacan et al (1977) compared the NPT characteristics of 11 impotent diabetic patients seeking evaluation for penile prosthesis, 11 age-matched impotent patients without known medical disorders, and a similar number of normal men. Diabetic men spent significantly less time in total erection and less time in full erection than the other two groups and also had significantly fewer episodes of maximum tumescence. Since the impotent diabetic group was selected on the basis of abnormal or absent nocturnal erections, it is not surprising that significant differences in NPT parameters were demonstrated. Subsequently, Karacan et al (1978) conducted an investigation of NPT in 35 impotent diabetic men, aged 33 to 70, and in 35 aged-matched controls. Diabetic patients, as a group, showed significant decreases in total penile tumescence time, duration and frequency of full erections and a reduction in the maximum increase in penile circumference. Within the diabetic group, 28 patients were considered organically impaired as evidenced by having less than one full penile tumescent episode per night. A full erection was operationally defined as a circumference increase, measured behind the glans, greater than or equal to 16 mm. This value is based on an estimate of 20 mm as the increase associated with full erection in normal men and on the assumption that an erection must be at least 80 per cent of maximum fullness to be effective for vaginal penetration. Hosking et al (1979) also employed absolute criteria in their study of 30 impotent diabetic patients in comparison with 11 healthy volunteers. Based on the observation that only six diabetic men and one control subject showed a maximum penile circumference increase of less than 15 mm (measured at the base), he concluded that in most diabetic patients impotence is due to psychological factors. Hosking et al noted a low correlation between evidence of peripheral and autonomic neuropathy and maximum penile circumference increases in diabetic patients. The studies of both Karacen et al and Hosking et al must be accepted with reservation because they used absolute criteria for defining full and partial erections. Because there are marked individual variations in penile circumference increases with full erection from 15 to 45 mm the practice of awakening the subjects on one of the experimental nights to obtain estimates of degree of erection, originally emphasized by Karacan, has become a necessity for optimal results (see below).

Fisher et al (1979) provided quantitative information on NPT in 30 impotent men including 12 diabetic patients evaluated during three study nights. Data was obtained on degree, duration, frequency and amount of nocturnal erectile episodes. Maximum tumescence was defined for each subject as 81 to 100 per cent of the greatest degree of tumescence estimated to be full by direct observation. If only partial tumescence was recorded, an estimate of potential maximum penile circumference was calculated based on a judgement of percentage of tumescence at the time of awakening. Patients were categorized as psychologically impotent on the basis of at least one maximum NPT episode of five minutes or more in duration per night. Frequency, degree, duration and amount of NPT were found to be significantly and markedly greater in the psychogenic group. It is of note that six mildly diabetic patients, originally thought to be suffering from psychogenic impotence based on detailed psychosexual evaluation, showed considerable NPT impairment and were reassigned, according to operational criteria, to the organically impotent group. Five diabetic patients exhibited briefly sustained full nocturnal erections averaging little more than two minutes of 'T max' (duration above 80 per cent of estimated full tumescence) per episode as against a mean duration of 11 minutes in the psychogenic group. In 15 to 20 per cent of the cases studied, NPT deficits were present in the apparent absence of organic causes, raising the possibility that, in at least some cases, NPT may be impaired for psychological reasons.

Recently Karacan (1980) assessed concurrently penile blood pressure, bulbocavernosus reflex response latency and plasma concentrations of testosterone and prolactin in 13 diabetic men with absent or abnormally

diminished nocturnal tumescence in an effort to identify possible patho-
genic determinants. In comparison with control data, the bulbocavernosus
response mean latency was significantly prolonged in the diabetic group and
penile systolic blood pressure was abnormally low in five patients.
Hormonal levels were within the normal range. Karacan concluded that
sacral neuropathy and vascular changes may play a significant role in the
pathogenesis of diabetic impotency and that the evaluation of penile blood
pressure and bulbocavernosus response latency should be considered in
diabetic patients with abnormal NPT recordings.

Validation studies

The need to validate NPT as a diagnostic method has been emphasized by
several investigators (Bancroft, 1980; Wasserman et al, 1980; Schiavi et al,
1981). Despite the increasing use of this procedure, there is only one report
on the diagnostic validity of the method. Marshall, Surridge and Delva
(1981) assigned, on the basis of medical history and psychiatric assessment,
independently of knowledge of NPT data, 27 impotent patients to one of
the following diagnostic categories: organic impotence, psychogenic
impotence, mixed aetiology and uncertain aetiology. NPT assessments were
conducted over two consecutive nights. A decision rule based on the
maximum erectile response observed for each patient (<11.5 mm $=$
organic; >11.5 mm $=$ psychogenic) led to the correct diagnosis in 80 per
cent of the cases. Accuracy was increased to 95 per cent when the decision
rule was based on the maximum frequency of nocturnal erections (two
episodes or less $=$ organic; three episodes or more $=$ psychogenic).
Replication on a different subject sample is required in order to confirm the
discriminating power of these criteria.

   In view of the importance of validating NPT as a diagnostic tool, we are
presently conducting a study on four age-matched groups: normal sexually
non-dysfunctional men, psychogenically impotent men, diabetic men
without sexual problems and impotent diabetic patients. The categorization
is made on the basis of extensive clinical evidence independent of NPT
information. Assignment to the psychogenic category is based on clear
evidence of psychological or relationship determinants, the selective or
situational nature of the erectile difficulties and no evidence of medical
illness. Diabetic subjects are divided into sexually functional and
dysfunctional groups. Assignment to the sexually dysfunctional group is
based on evidence of a temporal relation between diabetes and the progressive and global development of erectile impotence and on lack of evidence
of psychological causation. At present we have analysed data on 44
subjects, 13 normal, 16 psychogenic and 15 diabetic men: nine without and
six with erectile problems (mean age of normals was 28, psychogenic
impotent 28.4, diabetic non-dysfunctional 30, and diabetic impotent 27.4).
All non-diabetic subjects were drug-free during the study. Diabetic patients
were taking insulin or other antidiabetic medication and were under good
metabolic control. All subjects were studied under similar conditions in the
sleep laboratory during three nights each for a total of 132 study nights.
EEG, eye movement, heart rate and penile tumescence were monitored

continuously through the night. Penile tumescence was measured by means of two strain gauges, one placed around the penis near the base and the other just below the corona of the glans. During the third night visual checks were carried out to ascertain rigidity in relation to the recorded increase in penile circumference.

There were no significant differences between the groups in mean sleep and REM duration, number of REM periods per night and percentage of sleep time spent in REM. Mean sleep time ranged across the groups from 384 to 415 minutes, with 3.8 to 4.3 REM periods per night. Figure 1 provides information on NPT frequency variables that discriminated significantly among groups. Diabetic impotent men had fewer mean episodes of tumescence per night (F = 4.8, df 3/40, $P < 0.01$), markedly fewer episodes of maximum tumescence (F = 4.6, df 30/40, $P < .01$) and fewer episodes of maximum tumescence relative to the number of REM periods per night (F = 3.1, df 3/40, $P < .05$).

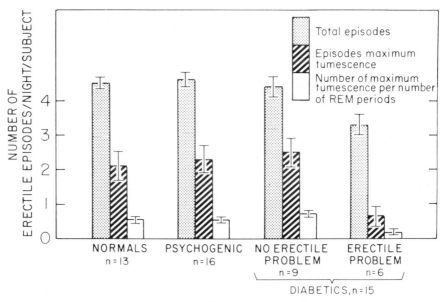

Figure 1. NPT frequency variables recorded over three study nights (mean ± SEM).

Figure 2 summarizes mean differences in duration parameters among the groups. Diabetic impotent men spent considerably less time in total tumescence per night, and significantly less time in maximum tumescence (F = 7.3, df 3/40, $P < 0.005$) and in simultaneous REM and tumescence (F = 2.9, df 3/40, $P < 0.05$) than the other three groups. There were no significant mean differences in frequency or duration variables among the normal, psychogenic and non-dysfunctional diabetics. Figures 3 to 6 demonstrate the pattern of NPT episodes and REM periods observed during a study night in a representative subject in each group. It can be seen that all sub-

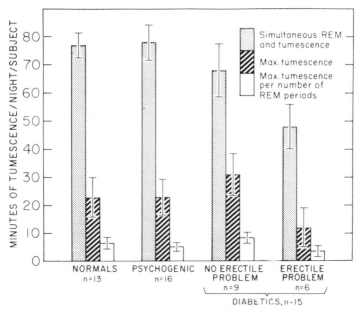

Figure 2. NPT duration variables recorded over three study nights (mean ± SEM).

jects show three to four REM periods per night and that each REM period is accompanied by a tumescent episode. The figures illustrate the wide range in tumescent patterns observed within and across subjects. The normal, psychogenically impotent and diabetic non-impotent subjects each show three episodes of maximum tumescence. Although the diabetically impotent men spent considerable sleep time in tumescence, none of the episodes reached the criterion for maximum tumescence.

Comparison of *mean group values* confirmed therefore the hypothesis that NPT recordings discriminate organically impotent diabetic men from non-dysfunctional diabetics, psychogenically impotent subjects and normal controls. The results also indicate that some NPT parameters such as total number of erectile episodes, frequency and duration of maximum tumescence and duration of simultaneous REM and tumescence are better able to effect such discrimination. Decision rules that may permit the accurate classification of *individual subjects* will be formulated after completing the study of an increased subject sample. It is important to mention that in all the groups a wide range of values was recorded for each measure, and that several normal and psychogenic men showed markedly decreased or absent maximum tumescent episodes during the three study nights.

Methodological considerations

Several theoretical and methodological issues stemming from the work previously reviewed merit discussion in order to clarify the diagnostic value of NPT assessments and to identify areas in need of investigation.

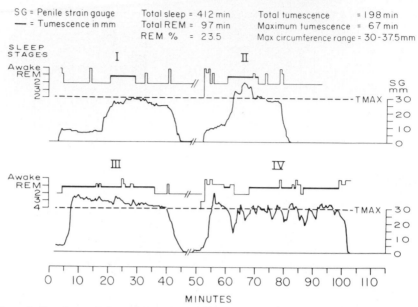

Figure 3. Erection cycle in a 27-year-old normal, non-dysfunctional, man showing three full erections during the second, third and fourth REM periods. Solid horizontal lines represent REM periods with Roman numerals indicating serial order from early in the night (I) to the end of the night (IV). The graph omits several hours of sleep when neither sleep nor tumescence were recorded. The same method of graphical presentation is used in Figures 4 to 6.

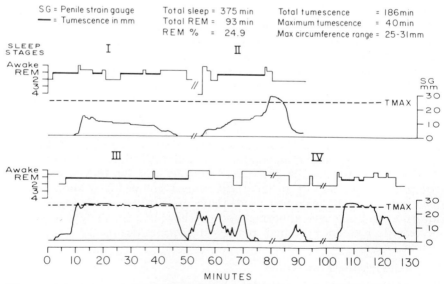

Figure 4. Thirty-one-year-old secondary impotent patient. The graph shows four REM periods accompanied by erections, three reaching maximum levels and one non-REM partial tumescent episode.

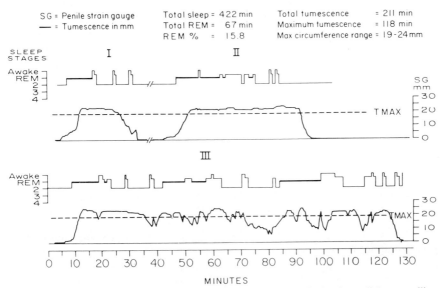

Figure 5. Twenty-six-year-old sexually non-dysfunctional man suffering from diabetes mellitus for the previous two years. The graph demonstrates three REM periods. The third one, interrupted by non-REM sleep, is considered a single episode because REM activity occurs at less than 30-minute intervals. All REM periods are accompanied by maximum tumescent episodes.

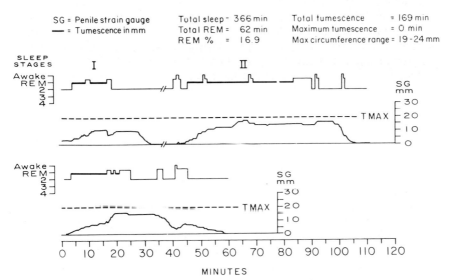

Figure 6. Twenty-nine-year-old man with diabetes mellitus since age 24 and a three-year history of erectile impotence. Considerable tumescent activity was recorded during the night, but none of the three REM-related episodes reached maximum levels of tumescence.

(a) The diagnostic significance of the method rests on the assumption that in psychogenically impotent men NPT is not impaired and, conversely, that normal NPT recordings rule out organic pathogenesis. Karacan et al are of the opinion that the existence of NPT impairment in about 20 per cent of patients, in the absence of known medical disorders, is due to covert organic factors. In keeping with this notion, Schmidt and Wise (1981) recently noted that seven out of 15 patients with secondary impotence without identifiable cause and impaired nocturnal penile tumescence had sleep-associated abnormalities such as frequent apnea and hypoventilation, myoclonus and a high incidence of bradycardia. The authors suggest that central nervous system abnormalities may play a significant aetiological role in some impotent patients in whom an organic cause cannot be identified. These data underline the value of concurrent EEG and psychophysiological monitoring in addition to penile tumescent recordings for the accurate interpretation of NPT data.

Fisher et al (1979) and Wasserman et al (1980) have speculated that psychological factors may play a significant role in the abnormal nocturnal penile patterns observed in some patients in whom medical disorders cannot be identified. Clinical evidence in support of this notion has been previously reported (Fisher et al, 1979); in the context of our ongoing validation study we have observed three normal non-dysfunctional men with markedly impaired NPT and two patients, categorized as psychogenically impotent, who did not exhibit a single full tumescent episode during the three study nights. These patients gained capacity for normal sexual function in response to sex therapy and/or psychotherapy and one of them, with primary impotence, remains potent one year after termination of treatment. In addition there is independent evidence suggesting that psychological factors may inhibit nocturnal penile tumescence. Fisher (1966) and Karacan et al (1966), as previously mentioned, both observed an inhibition of penile tumescent episodes in normal men during REM periods associated with dreams of high anxiety content. Some (Jovanović, 1969), but not all, investigators (Fisher et al, 1979) have reported a decrease in nocturnal erectile activity during the first study night, presumably due to stressful aspects in the recording situation. In the context of sleep-hormonal studies conducted in our laboratories we have also noted a modest, but significant, impairment in some NPT parameters independent of sleep disturbance during nights when sequential blood sampling are conducted. Emotional disorders such as depression may also significantly influence nocturnal tumescent activity. Jovanović (1972) and Roose et al (1981), for instance, have presented data indicating that in some men suffering from severe depression NPT was absent or markedly impaired. In the studies of Roose et al recovery from depression in two subjects was accompanied by re-establishment of sexual competency and normalization of NPT.

The psychological effects of the laboratory situation, the experimental procedures and the relationship between the subject and the night technician on NPT measures have not been evaluated. These factors may produce anxiety or other dysphoric affects, such as shame and embarrassment in connection with exposure of the penis and being awakened and examined at night, and may have an inhibiting effect on erection, preventing full tumescence. It will be necessary to apply psychological testing instruments for anxiety and other affects and also to observe more carefully during sleep the physiological concomitants of anxiety, such as heart and respiratory rates. With portable NPT monitors it may also be possible to develop an adequate method of procedure at home and in this way avoid the laboratory situation. Unfortunately, at present, home monitors appear to be applied inappropriately (see below).

The possibility that NPT may not be impaired in some cases where organic factors are pathogenically involved in erectile impotence should also be considered. Since the degree of overlapping between the neurophysiological and endocrine mechanisms that subserve erotically-induced and REM-related erections is not known, it is at least theoretically possible that some subjects may exhibit normal NPT and yet have abnormalities in the physiological substrates that mediate sexual arousal.

(b) As mentioned above, there are considerable interindividual variations in penile circumference increases associated with full tumescence. The existence of individual differences that range from 15 to 45 mm measured at the base of the penis and from 10 to 48 mm behind the glans necessitates visual checks to ascertain the amount of increase in circumference associated with full tumescence. This method provides direct information when full tumescent episodes are observed but is of questionable validity in organically impaired patients who do not attain maximum erectile capacity. In these instances, estimates of full erection may be obtained by extrapolation from observations of partial erections. This calculation presupposes, however, a linear relation between circumference increase and penile rigidity, an assumption that is open to question.

Limited information exists on the relation between penile circumference and rigidity. Recently, Metz and Wagner (1981) approached this question experimentally by recording simultaneously penile circumference and intracavernous pressure during artificial erection, produced by saline infusion into the corpora cavernosa of six fresh cadavers. They noted that circumferential changes reached maximum levels at pressures within the corpora cavernosa below those required to achieve full erection. Godec and Cass (1981) devised an analogue model for the study of the relation between penile expansion and rigidity, from which they derived a clinical evaluation method. They measured penile circumference changes associated with full erections produced acutely in impotent patients by saline infusion into the corpora cavernosa. The degree of circumference increase associated with penile rigidity in this test provided a reference point for interpretation of tumescent changes during nocturnal erections. The authors noted that above a certain intracavernosus pressure changes in penile expansion no longer parallel intracavernosus pressure but, in contrast to the findings of Metz and Wagner, they observed continued increases in penile circumference after the levelling of intracorporeal pressure. It is obvious from this research that the relation between penile circumference, rigidity and intracavernosus pressure requires further study. The clinical importance of this issue has recently been emphasized by Wein et al (1981) who observed that of 134 patients who underwent NPT evaluation, 23 had increases in penile circumference within normal ranges but without sufficient rigidity to effect vaginal penetration. A procedure that monitors changes in penile rigidity with minimal interference of erectile activity and sleep, under development in several laboratories, would constitute a significant methodological advance. In the meantime, adequate evaluation requires systematic awakenings during episodes of maximum penile expansion and direct observations and examination by a trained observer.

(c) There is a need to conduct parametric studies in order to identify the most valid, reliable and sensitive NPT variables indicative of organic erectile impairment and to formulate decision rules that best discriminate among clinical groups. At present it is not certain whether central nervous system dysfunction, general metabolic disorders or hormonal abnormalities affect NPT, but it would be premature to assume that these conditions have the same effect on NPT measures as peripheral neurovascular pathology. This is an empirical issue likely to be resolved only by systematic studies that compare EEG and NPT variables across age-matched diagnostic groups.

CLINICAL APPLICATION OF THE METHOD

In view of the increasing use of NPT monitoring for differential diagnosis of erectile disorders, it seems important to emphasize the relevance of several procedural aspects for a correct interpretation of results.

1. *Recording variables.* Recordings of EEG and electro-oculographic variables, although demanding of time and specific skills, are essential to determine the extent to which NPT abnormalities may reflect impaired sleep patterns or disturbed CNS activity. In addition, the measuring of penile tumescence by means of two strain gauge loops placed at the base and behind the glans of the penis can be valuable in the detection of possible pathology such as covert genital defects or Peyronie's disease.

2. *Number of nights.* At least two study nights are necessary to adequately characterize NPT function in most subjects. As stated previously, sleep and NPT patterns may be impaired during the first recording night in individuals who require habituation to the procedure. Patients are studied in our laboratories during three nights; following two nights of undisturbed sleep, systematic awakenings are conducted during the third night for the assessment of penile rigidity.

3. *Assessment of penile rigidity.* The importance of not relying solely on circumferential changes for the assessment of erectile capacity has been emphasized previously. In the absence of a direct method of monitoring penile rigidity without disturbing sleep, systematic awakenings during erectile episodes need to be carried out for estimation by subject and investigator of degree of rigidity. This procedure is complicated by the difficulty of properly timing awakenings and of estimating full erections from observation of partial erections in organically impotent patients. A

complementary approach which we have occasionally found helpful in estimating the relation between circumferential change and penile rigidity is based on penile strain gauge recordings in relation to direct observations carried out while the subjects masturbate in the laboratory. Photographic recordings of erection and the use of a device developed by Karacan to measure the 'buckling pressure' of the penis provides additional approaches to document erectile capacity. According to Karacan's use of this method, penile rigidity that buckles under a pressure of less than 60 mm Hg is considered insufficient for vaginal penetration. Pressures above 100 mm Hg are considered indicative of sufficient rigidity for intromission. No data has yet been presented to support the validity of the observations derived by this buckling device.

4. *Criteria for diagnostic assignments.* Since no uniform criteria have evolved, NPT recordings are presently interpreted in an idiosyncratic manner, preventing meaningful comparison of results across laboratories. Wasserman et al (1980), following a critical evaluation of NPT criteria used by different investigators, suggests that diagnostic decisions should be based on the demonstration of erectile capacity of sufficient rigidity and duration for satisfactory intercourse rather than on comparisons with age-matched normal subjects. These investigators categorize patients as 'psychogenically impotent' when they have at least one full erection, lasting for five consecutive minutes during three nights, which is confirmed by observation to be adequate for intromission. Although the five-minute period might be long enough for intercourse it does not differentiate deteriorating organic cases such as diabetics who may have one or two erections of that length in a general picture of erectile devastation. For clinical purposes we currently require a mean frequency of one full erection per night in order to categorize a patient as psychogenically impotent. This criterion is, however, arbitrary and in need of systematic evaluation. (For a detailed description of our methods of procedure and data analysis see Fisher et al, 1979.)

During the last few years several portable devices have been developed for the recording of NPT with the aim of simplifying the assessment process and rendering it less costly (Bohlen, 1981). Because of the increasing and, at times, indiscriminate use of these devices, a note of caution seems appropriate. The gathering of valid information rests on: (1) Adequate understanding by the patient of the use of the monitoring equipment. This includes proper calibration to insure that accurate calculation of penile circumference can be made from the record. (2) Assessment during at least two nights to permit habituation to the recording procedure. (3) Reasonable certainty that the sleep pattern is not disturbed. (4) No medication, drugs or alcohol intake that may influence the nocturnal penile activity. (5) Direct observation of penile rigidity relative to recordings of circumference change. Some new monitoring instruments contain for this purpose a sound signalling system that is triggered when the increase in penile circumference reaches a predetermined criterion level. In addition to the patient, an independent observer should provide a rigidity estimate since subjective assessments obtained during induced awakenings in the night can be grossly inaccurate. Since most of these conditions are difficult to achieve or control outside the laboratory considerable caution should be exercised in the interpretation of NPT data recorded in the subject's home.

CONCLUSIONS

The frequent association of psychological and organic factors in the pathogenesis of erectile impotence in diabetic patients creates difficult problems of differential diagnosis. A detailed psychosexual history is particularly helpful in exploring the aetiological significance of psychological factors but is less helpful in determining the extent of organic deficit in erectile capacity. The medical history and laboratory studies may establish the existence of a coexisting illness such as diabetes but do not demonstrate its causal relation to the sexual disorder. The monitoring of NPT is a new method that offers promise of objectively assessing organic impairment in diabetes as well as in other illness that affect sexual functioning. Several methodological issues are of critical importance for a correct interpretation of NPT results. Further research is required in order to validate and better delineate the clinical applicability of the method. At the present state of development, this procedure should be used cautiously and in the context of a thorough clinical evaluation.

ACKNOWLEDGEMENTS

This article is based in part on research supported by USPHS research grants MH 27513 and AM 20845 and by the New Land Foundation.

REFERENCES

Abelson, D. (1975) Diagnostic value of the penile pulse and blood pressure: a doppler study of impotence in diabetics. *Journal of Urology,* 113, 636-639.

Aserinsky, E. & Kleitman, N. (1955) A motility cycle in sleeping infants as manifested by ocular and gross bodily activity. *Journal of Applied Physiology,* 8, 11-18.

Bancroft, J. (1980) Diabetic impotence (letter to editor). *British Medical Journal,* i, 11-18.

Bohlen, J. (1981) Sleep erection monitoring in the evaluation of male erectile failure. *Urologic Clinics of North America,* 8, 119-134.

Buck, A. C., Reed, P. I., Siddiq, Y. K., Chisholm, G. D. & Fraser, R. (1976) Bladder dysfunction and neuropathy in diabetes. *Diabetologia,* 12, 251-258.

Ellenberg, M. (1971) Impotence in diabetes: the neurologic factor. *Annals of Internal Medicine,* 75, 213-219.

Ewing, D. J., Campbell, I. W. & Clarke, B. F. (1976) Mortality and diabetic autonomic neuropathy. *Lancet,* i, 601-603.

Faerman, I., Vilar, O., Rivarola, M. A., Rosner, J. M., Jadzinsky, M. N., Fox, D., Perez-Lloret, A., Bernstein-Hahn, L. & Saraceni, D. (1972) Impotence and diabetes: study of androgenic function in diabetic impotent males. *Diabetes,* 21, 23-30.

Fisher, C. (1966) Dreaming and sexuality. In *Psychoanalysis — A General Psychology: Essays in Honor of Heinz Hartman* (Ed.) Loewenstein, R. M., Newman, L. M. & Schur, M. pp. 537-563. New York: International University Press.

Fisher, C., Gross, J. & Zuch, J. (1964) A preliminary report on a cycle of penile erection synchronous with REM sleep. *Fourth Annual Meeting of the Association for the Psychophysiological Study of Sleep. Palo Alto, Calif.*

Fisher, C., Gross, J. & Zuch, J. (1965) Cycle of penile erection synchronous with dreaming (REM) sleep. *Archives of General Psychiatry,* **12,** 29-45.

Fisher, C., Schiavi, R. C., Lear, H., Edwards, A., Davis, D. M. & Witkin, A. P. (1975) The assessment of nocturnal REM erections in the differential diagnosis of sexual impotence. *Journal of Sex and Marital Therapy,* **1,** 277-289.

Fisher, C., Schiavi, R. C., Edwards, A., Davis, D. M., Reitman, M. & Fine, J. (1979) Evaluation of nocturnal penile tumescence in the differential diagnosis of sexual impotence. *Archives of General Psychiatry,* **36,** 431-437.

Godec, C. J. & Cass, A. S. (1981) Quantification of erection. *Journal of Urology,* **126,** 345-347.

Hosking, D. J., Bennet, T., Hampton, J. R., Evans, D. F., Clark, A. J. & Robertson, G. (1979) Diabetic impotence: studies of nocturnal erection during REM sleep, *British Medical Journal,* **ii,** 1394-1396.

Hursch, C. J., Karacan, I. & Williams, R. L. (1972) Some characteristics of nocturnal penile tumescence in early middle-aged males. *Comprehensive Psychiatry,* **13,** 539-548.

Jovanović, U. J. (1972) Sexuelle reaktionen und schlafperiodik bei menschen: Ergebnisse experimenteller untersuchungen. *Beitrage fur Sexualforschung,* **51,** 1-292.

Jovanović, V. J. (1969) Der effekt der ersten untersuchungsnacht auf die erektionen im schlaf. *Psychotherapy and Psychosomatics,* **17,** 295-308.

Jovanović, V. J. & Tan-eli, B. (1969) Penile erections during sleep. *Arzneimittel-Forschung,* **19,** 966-974.

Khan, E. & Fisher, C. (1969) The sleep characteristics of the normal aged male. *Journal of Nervous and Mental Disease,* **148,** 477-494.

Karacan, I. (1970) Clinical value of nocturnal erection in the prognosis and diagnosis of impotence. *Medical Aspects of Human Sexuality,* April Issue, 27-34.

Karacan, I. (1980) Diagnosis of erectile impotence in diabetes mellitus. *Annals of Internal Medicine,* **92,** 334-337.

Karacan, I., Goodenough, D. R., Shapiro, A. & Starker, S. (1966) Erection cycle during sleep in relation to dream anxiety. *Archives of General Psychiatry,* **15,** 183-189.

Karacan, I., Hursch, C. J., Williams, R. L. & Littell, R. C. (1972a) Some characteristics of nocturnal penile tumescence during puberty. *Pediatric Research,* **6,** 529-537.

Karacan, I., Hursch, C. J., Williams, R. L. & Thornby, J. I. (1972b) Some characteristics of nocturnal penile tumescence in young adults. *Archives of General Psychiatry,* **26,** 351-356.

Karacan, I., Williams, R. L., Thornby, J. I. & Salis, P. J. (1975) Sleep-related penile tumescence as a function of age. *American Journal of Psychiatry,* **132,** 932-937.

Karacan, I., Salis, P. J., Thornby, J. I. & Williams, R. L. (1976) The ontogeny of nocturnal penile tumescence. *Waking and Sleeping,* **1,** 27-44.

Karacan, I., Scott, F. B., Salis, P. J., Attia, S. L., Ware, J. C., Altinel, A. & Williams, R. L. (1977) Nocturnal erections, differential diagnosis of impotence and diabetes. *Biological Psychiatry,* **12,** 373-380.

Karacan, I., Salis, P. J., Ware, J. C., Dervent, B., Williams, R. L., Scott, F. B., Attia, S. L. & Beutler, L. E. (1978) Nocturnal penile tumescence and diagnosis in diabetic impotence. *American Journal of Psychiatry,* **135,** 191-197.

Marshall, P., Surridge, D. M. & Delva, N. (1981) The role of nocturnal penile tumescence in differentiating between organic and psychogenic impotence: the first stage of validation. *Archives of Sexual Behavior,* **10,** 1-10.

Metz, P. & Wagner, G. N. (1981) Penile circumference and erection. *Urology,* **28,** 268-270.

Ohlmeyer, P., Brilmayer, H. & Hüllstrung, H. (1944) Periodische Vorgange im Schlaf. *Pflugers Archiv,* **248,** 559-560.

Rastogi, G. K., Chakraborti, J. & Sinha, M. K. (1974) Serum gonadotrophins (LH and FSH) and their response to synthetic LHRH in diabetic men with and without impotence. *Hormonal and Metabolic Research,* **6,** 335-336.

Roose, S. P., Glassman, A. H., Walsh, B. T. & Cullen, K. (1981) Reversible loss of nocturnal penile tumescence during depression. Paper presented at *American Psychiatric Association Meeting, New Orleans.*

Schiavi, R. C. & Hogan, B. (1979) Sexual problems in diabetes mellitus: psychological aspects. *Diabetes Care,* **2,** 9-17.

Schiavi, R. C., Fisher, C., Quadland, M. & Gloger, T. (1981) The diagnosis of erectile disorders. In *Exerpta Medica. Proceedings 5th World Congress of Sexology* (Ed.) Hoch, Z. & Lief, H. I. (in press).

Schmidt, H. S. & Wise, H. A. (1981) Significance of impaired penile tumescence and associated polysomnographic abnormalities in the impotent patient. *Journal of Urology,* **126,** 348-351.

Wasserman, M. D., Pollak, C. P., Spielman, A. J. & Weitzman, E. D. (1980) Theoretical and technical problems in the measurement of nocturnal penile tumescence for the differential diagnosis of impotence. *Psychosomatic Medicine,* **42,** 575-585.

Wein, A. J., Fishkin, R., Carpiniello, V. L. & Malloy, T. R. (1981) Expansion without significant rigidity during nocturnal penile tumescence testing. A potential source of misinterpretation. *Journal of Urology,* **126,** 343-344.

11

Sexuality of Diabetic Women

JOHN BANCROFT

The sexual problems of diabetic women have received much less attention than those of diabetic men. One possible reason for this neglect is a simple fact that the sexuality of women is less affected by diabetes and they are therefore less likely to present sexual problems to the clinician. As we shall see, recent evidence supports this view. But if it is confirmed, it will be of some importance to understand why female diabetics are so different from male diabetics in this respect. In general, male/female differences in sexuality and sexual dysfunction are fruitful areas for study.

In this chapter the limited evidence from female diabetics will be briefly reviewed and possible explanations for the observed male/female differences considered.

EARLY STUDIES

In 1971, Kolodny reported a comparison of 125 diabetic and 100 non-diabetic women. Both groups were interviewed during hospitalization, the reasons for which were not given, though the control group had 'primary illness of at least 3 months' duration'.

The two groups did not differ in frequency of sexual intercourse, level of sexual interest, incidence of dyspareunia or impairment of vaginal lubrication. They did differ, however, in their experience of orgasm. A complete absence of orgasm during the preceding year was reported by 35.2 per cent of the diabetic women, compared with 6 per cent of the controls ($P = < 0.01$). In addition, all of the non-orgasmic control women had *never* previously experienced orgasm, whereas in all but four of the non-orgasmic diabetic women, orgasms had been experienced at some previous stage. This orgasmic dysfunction was related to the duration of the diabetes, but not to age, severity of diabetes, insulin requirements or the presence of diabetic complications.

Ellenberg (1977) studied 100 diabetic women, 54 of whom had neuropathy, either autonomic, peripheral or both. The incidence of orgasmic difficulty was 18 per cent, which Ellenberg concluded was no different to other studies of orgasmic function in normal women. The lack of any appropriate group for comparison, however, makes such conclusions of

Clinics in Endocrinology and Metabolism — Vol. 11, No. 3, November 1982.
0300-595X/82/11.03/785 $03.00 © 1982 W. B. Saunders Company Ltd

doubtful value. Of more relevance is the comparison between women with and those without evidence of neuropathy. Here the results were negative. The existence of neuropathy, even when producing severe autonomic disturbances, was not apparently associated with obvious sexual impairment. Two other studies (Montenero, Donatone and Magi, 1973; Zrustova, Rostlapil and Kabrhelová, 1978) reported an increased incidence of sexual difficulties in diabetic women, but in neither study was there a satisfactory control group and these conclusions are also of uncertain validity.

RECENT EVIDENCE

Two recent studies, involving control groups, have both reached very similar conclusions. Jensen (1981) studied 80 diabetic women and 80 diabetic men attending outpatient clinics and compared them with 40 women and 40 men attending their general practitioners' surgeries, excluding those with any kind of chronic somatic disease or previous psychiatric treatment. The male diabetics reported an incidence of sexual dysfunction similar to that in other studies (see Chapter 9) and significantly greater than the control men and both groups of women. The diabetic and control women did not differ from each other in reported sexual dysfunction (27.5 per cent and 25 per cent respectively). Reduced libido was the commonest complaint (24 per cent and 23 per cent respectively). Orgasmic dysfunction was reported by 11 per cent of the diabetic and 7.5 per cent of the control women. Significantly more diabetic women reported reduced vaginal lubrication (24 per cent and 8 per cent respectively, $P = < 0.05$) though they did not differ from controls in the incidence of dyspareunia (10 per cent and 8 per cent respectively). Diabetic women with peripheral neuropathy were more likely than those without to report sexual dysfunction (44 per cent and 20 per cent respectively).

Tyrer et al (1982) compared 82 diabetic women attending a diabetic out-patient department with 47 'normal' women attending a family planning clinic and selected by the clinic doctors as having no obvious sexual problem. Each woman was assessed using interview-based ratings of various aspects of sexual function, as well as a variety of pencil and paper measures of sexual attitudes and attitudes towards the husband.

The diabetic women differed in their contraceptive usage, a reminder that diabetes does pose special problems affecting fertility as well as contraception (Steele and Duncan, 1980). But apart from this, the comparison showed no obvious sexual disadvantages for the diabetic women. They were certainly no different in terms of orgasmic function or sexual interest. They were more variable in their vaginal response to sexual stimulation (i.e., lubrication), being more likely to report either good or poor responses, whereas the responses of controls were more often in the intermediate part of the range. The diabetic women reported significantly fewer *negative* feelings during sexual activity.

There were also differences in the women's appraisal of themselves and their partners. Using a semantic differential (Whitehead and Mathews, 1976) the diabetic women rated themselves and their male partners significantly less 'potent' than did the control women. Potency, in this sense, is not sexual but more related to strength and activity. Twenty-one per cent of the diabetic women believed that their diabetes had had a beneficial effect on their marriage (mainly because their husbands showed more concern), compared with nine per cent who felt it had been detrimental.

A subgroup of the diabetic women ($n = 58$) and controls ($n = 44$) also completed the Sexual Experience Scale of Frenken (1976) covering 'sexual motivation' and 'attraction to marriage'. The two groups did not differ in either scale (sexual motivation scale: Diabetics 43.6 ($\pm$ 7.3), controls 45.2 ($\pm$7.6) NS; 'attraction to marriage' scale: diabetics 77.6 ($\pm$8.3), controls 76.2 ($\pm$8.6) NS.

Whilst these findings reinforce the sexual similarity of the two groups, they do not provide any further evidence of differences in the marriages. However, it remains an interesting possibility that diabetes produces particular effects on marriage and more appropriate measures may be required before this question can be properly answered.

Each of the diabetic women was assessed for evidence of autonomic neuropathy by objective clinical tests as well as by enquiry of symptoms. They were categorized as being normal, 'borderline' (i.e., abnormal tests but no symptoms) and 'symptomatic' (i.e., abnormal tests and symptoms). Sixty-two per cent were normal, 20 per cent were borderline and 18 per cent were symptomatic. Comparison of these three groups showed no differences in any of the measures of sexual function, except for a non-significant tendency for those women with no autonomic neuropathy to show stronger non-genital arousal during sexual activity.

SEXUAL FUNCTION IN DIABETICS: MALE—FEMALE DIFFERENCES

Obviously in assessing sexual function, particularly in women, it is important to have an appropriate control group who are assessed in a similar way. In this respect, we should confine our attention to the studies by Kolodny (1971), Jensen (1981) and Tyrer et al (1982), and when considering the effects of autonomic neuropathy those of Ellenberg (1977) and Tyrer et al (1982).

The two studies by Jensen and Tyrer et al are strikingly similar to one another in their findings, though the method of assessing sexual function was less detailed and thorough in the former study. Both, however, are discrepant with the findings of Kolodny. The explanation for this difference is not clear. Control of diabetes may be an important factor. Poor control not only may lead to general debility and secondary non-specific sexual effects, but also will increase the likelihood of vaginal infection and pruritus. The degree of diabetic control of the woman in Kolodny's study is not stated, but the fact that they had all been hospitalized increases the likelihood that they had been through a period of poor control. In the two later studies, involving routine out-patient attenders, good diabetic control can be assumed.

If we accept the conclusion of the two most recent studies, that diabetic women are not prone to sexual impairment, then we are faced with a striking difference between female and male diabetics. In the case of the male, erectile failure is a common sexual consequence of diabetes. As reviewed in Chapter 9, this is likely to be due to either autonomic neuropathy, angiopathy, or both, plus the almost inevitable added effect of anxiety and other psychological factors.

The comparable physiological responses in the female are vaginal lubrication, which is believed to result from the vasocongestion of the vaginal wall, together with tumescence of the vulva and clitoris. Both recent studies report some evidence of impairment in this respect. Whilst all of these genital responses contribute to satisfactory vaginal intercourse, none is essential or irreplaceable. By contrast, vaginal entry with anything less than a full erection in the male is difficult. Erection for the man is thus effectively an all or nothing phenomenon — if the required rigidity is not reached, the accompanying anxiety may be quite sufficient to produce a more limited erection than would otherwise have occurred.

Whereas male diabetics quite commonly report an alteration of the emission process (Fairburn et al, 1982) and occasionally experience retrograde ejaculation, there is no evidence that orgasm *per se* is affected by diabetes. Orgasm, as distinct from seminal emission, remains a neurophysiological mystery, but it probably involves the same mechanisms in men and women. If orgasm is not affected in male diabetics, why should it be so in female diabetics? According to Jensen and Tyrer et al it is not. Kolodny's earlier findings therefore remain difficult to explain.

In women, orgasm should be seen as part of the total sexual experience and if other aspects are impaired (e.g., leading to no enjoyment or reduced arousal) then orgasm may also suffer. Orgasmic dysfunction may therefore be part of a consistent pattern of sexual unresponsiveness, as distinct from a localized or discrete dysfunction (Bancroft, Tyrer and Warner, 1982). It is not clear from Kolodny's report which of these applied in his women, though general unresponsiveness did not seem to be present. In contrast to the male, the effects of any minimal physiological impairment in women may be determined much more by other aspects of the sexual relationship. Thus it is worth speculating that in diabetic women other psychological consequences of the diabetes, affecting the quality of the relationship in a positive way, may counteract the relatively minor negative physiological effects of the diabetes. In order to pursue this possibility, it will be necessary to study in more detail the marriages of diabetic women to see whether they differ in any consistent way with non-diabetic marriages. It is also possible that the marriages of diabetic men may have a different effect on their sexuality. Whereas the diabetic woman may feel more tender and caring towards her husband because he is supportive with her diabetes, the diabetic man may find that his dependence on his wife undermines his sense of masculinity and has negative repercussions on his sexuality. Further evidence of the quality of marriages for male and female diabetics may throw further light on this issue.

CONCLUSIONS

At the present time, the weight of evidence suggests that female diabetics with good diabetic control are relatively free from sexual impairment, even when they have severe autonomic neuropathy. This is in striking contrast with the male diabetic, who has a high incidence of erectile difficulties, and often disturbances of ejaculatory function. These are very clearly associated with autonomic neuropathy.

It has been postulated that the sexuality of women is more determined by interpersonal factors than that of men and that the interpersonal consequences of diabetes differ for the diabetic woman and for the diabetic man. Whilst such factors may be contributing to the striking sex differences of sexual dysfunction that are being reported, other possible explanations should be considered. It is possible, for example, that the autonomic nervous system may play a very different role in the sexuality of women and men. At the present time, it is appropriate to keep an open mind on these issues.

REFERENCES

Bancroft, J., Tyrer, G. & Warner, P. (1982) The assessment of sexual problems in women. *British Journal of Sexual Medicine,* **9** (81), 30-37.

Ellenberg, M. (1977) Sexual aspects of the female diabetic. *Mount Sinai Journal of Medicine,* **44,** 495-500.

Fairburn, C. G., Wu, F. C., McCulloch, D. K., Borsay, D. Q., Ewing, D. J., Clarke, B. F. & Bancroft, J. (1982) The clinical features of diabetic impotence: a preliminary study. *British Journal of Psychiatry,* **140,** 447-452.

Frenken, J. (1976) Afkeer van seksualiteit. Van Loghum, Slaterus-Deventer. (English summary pp. 219-225.)

Jensen, S. B. (1981) Diabetic sexual dysfunction: a comparative study of 160 insulin treated diabetic men and women and an age-matched control group. *Archives of Sexual Behavior,* **10,** 493-504.

Kolodny, R. C. (1971) Sexual dysfunction in diabetic females. *Diabetes,* **20,** 557-559.

Montenero, P., Donatone, E. & Magi, D. (1973) Diabète et activité sexuelle chez la femme. *Journal Annelles Diabetologie de L'Hotel-Dieu,* **11-13,** 91-103.

Steele, J. M. & Duncan, L. J. P. (1980) Contraception for the insulin dependent diabetic. *Diabetes Care,* **3,** 557-560.

Tyrer, G., Steele, J. M., Ewing, D. J., Bancroft, J., Warner, P. & Clarke, B. F. (1982) Sexual responsiveness in diabetic women. (Submitted for publication.)

Whitehead, A. & Mathews, A. (1976) Attitude change during behavioural treatment of sexual inadequacy. *British Journal of Social and Clinical Psychology,* **16,** 275-281.

Zrustová, M., Rostlapil, J. & Kabrhelová, A. (1978) Sexualři poruchy u zen S úplavici cukrovou Cs. *Gynekologie,* **43,** 277-280.

Index

Note: Page numbers of chapter titles are in **bold face** type.